CHINESE HERBAL MEDICINE

FOR BEGINNERS

Advanced Methods and Remedies to Cure Different Ailments and Health Problems with Chinese Herbal Medicine

JESSICA CHONG

Table of Contents

Introduction

Traditional Chinese Medicine is a medical system that has treated people and alleviated their pain for millennia. Even with the rise of technology and numerous scientific breakthroughs over the years, you'd be surprised to learn that TCM has undergone very few changes since its development.

The core of TCM is Qi, the vital life force that travels through the body. If Qi becomes subject to any imbalance, it can result in illness. These imbalances are triggered by changes in the yin and yang, the two harmonious yet opposing forces that make up the vital life force.

The theory behind this holistic healing system is that humans are nothing but microcosms in a humungous universe, making us inherently connected to nature and affected by its forces. Since yin and yang represent the balance between any two opposing forces in the universe, the balance between illness and health is also a core TCM concept. Therefore, this medical system aims to restore each person's health and disease balance through treatments.

You have to strive for a balance between the organs in your body and the elements of metal, earth, wood, water, and fire to regain your internal balance. The most popular treatments of TCM include acupuncture, cupping, tai chi, moxibustion, massage, and herbal remedies.

The dynamics of the modern-day world have made us subject to ongoing stress and pressure. Of course, this hinders our internal balance, making us less attuned to nature, and affecting our mental, emotional, physical, and spiritual health. So, seeking holistic medicine approaches, like TCM, and gaining a deeper understanding is as important today as ever. Very few people realize the importance of practicing holistic Medicine even when they don't have any symptoms. The best thing about these wellness programs is that they're healing and preventative.

Traditional Chinese Medicine is a natural yet highly effective approach that addresses the root causes of illnesses. Unlike over-the-counter medicines, TCM doesn't merely mask or alleviate the symptoms because it fixes the trigger behind the disease. Its effects are very lasting, allowing us to stay balanced. TCM also encourages your body to self-heal, as it brings balance to your inner systems, boosts the health of your vital organs, improves your immunity, raises your energy labels, diminishes stress and anxiety, alleviates pain, and keeps several pre-existing illnesses from progressing.

This book is a comprehensive beginner's guide to traditional Chinese Medicine. You will find everything you need to know about advanced methods and remedies to cure different health conditions and ailments with several TCM methods. After reading this book, you'll have an in-depth understanding of traditional Chinese Medicine, its philosophies, and its different diagnostic methods. You'll also learn cupping, gua sha, moxibustion, and

Chinese Herbology, their benefits, and how to practice them. This guide walks you through the different remedies in TCM and provides practical solutions for managing anxiety, illness, and pain. This book includes step-by-step instructions on safely and effectively using these treatments.

So, start your journey of restoring your health naturally with Chinese Herbal Medicine.

Chapter 1

Traditional Chinese Medicine

If you're looking for an alternative system of Medicine for your health concerns, Traditional Chinese Medicine is one of the most popular options. However, many people are concerned about trying alternative medical systems without knowing what that system entails.

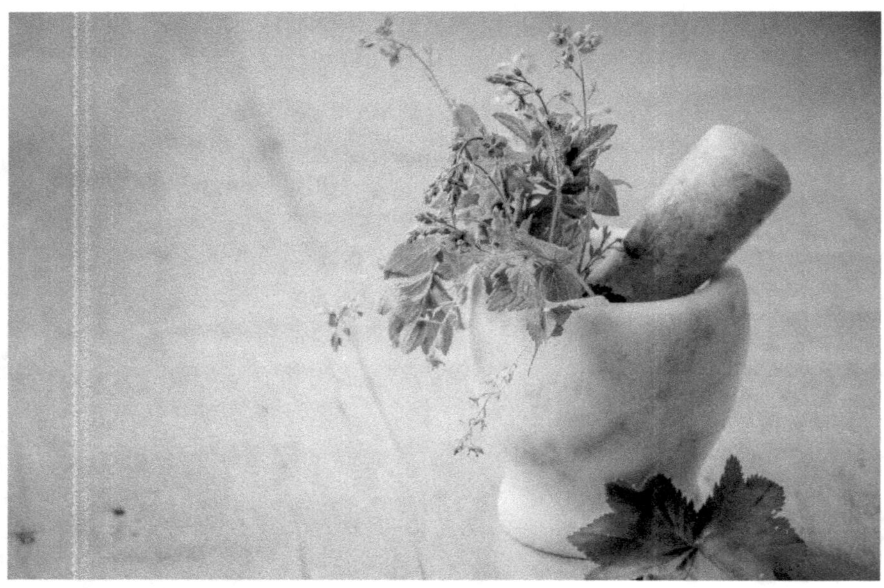

Despite its popularity, many people remain uninformed about Traditional Chinese Medicine (TCM). This book will help you understand what this medical system involves and offer DIY recipes and herbal medications you can use at home.

However, before you explore DIY options, it's essential to understand what TCM involves, its history, and its branches.

Understanding Traditional Chinese Medicine

As its name implies, Traditional Chinese Medicine (TCM) is an alternative medical practice used in China for thousands of years.

The most important aspect of understanding TCM is Qi or Chi. In essence, Qi is a universal energy source sometimes considered to be the vital force of life. Every human possesses Qi in their bodies, and a balanced Qi is essential for good health and happiness.

Qi cannot be destroyed; however, it can transform from one aspect to another (yin and yang). Each aspect must be balanced. It can result in physical and emotional illnesses if they are imbalanced. TCM aims to bring the levels of Qi in a person's body back into balance.

While Western allopathic medication aims to treat a person's physical symptoms, TCM concerns a person's holistic well-being.

Several practices are used in TCM, including:

- Qigong
- Acupuncture

- Acupressure

- Moxibustion

- Yin and Yang

- Herbology

- Cupping

- Tai Chi

While many people are skeptical about the effects of TCM, scientific evidence shows that many of these practices have value. For example, acupuncture and acupressure are commonly accepted practices for treating chronic pain.

Additionally, many herbs used in Chinese Herbology have been scientifically proven to have healing properties. Tai chi has been shown to improve balance, and cupping is effective for pain relief.

The main aspect to consider when practicing TCM is that no matter which practice you indulge in, your practitioner should be experienced and educated. Using uneducated practitioners for practices like cupping and acupuncture can be dangerous.

The primary challenge with Chinese Herbology is the lack of FDA approval. However, if you work with someone with experience and education, who knows what they are doing, there shouldn't be any risk.

Additionally, TCM should be used as a complementary practice. Many TCM practitioners will give you this advice – it should not be used as a replacement for traditional medication. Always consult your medical professional before engaging in any TCM activities.

It is especially true if you're considering Chinese Herbology and taking medications. Some herbs might negatively interact with medications, and it's essential that you and your TCM practitioner know what to expect. For the same reason, always be upfront with your TCM practitioner and medical professional about the medications you're taking and alternative therapies you're benefitting from. It allows all professionals treating you to adjust their therapies so they don't conflict with each other.

History of Traditional Chinese Medicine

Traditional Chinese Medicine can trace its roots back 3000 years to the Shang dynasty. Archeologists and historians found that the first concepts of therapeutic activities were during the Shang dynasty (14th-11th centuries BC).

However, these therapeutic activities have little resemblance to modern TCM. There is no evidence that the Shang dynasty's people's conception of illness was as we understand it today. When they suffered an illness, it was brought on by the ancestors' spirits, and there was little understanding of germ theory or bodily imbalances causing sickness. They did not use Herbology as part of their therapeutic treatments.

Although, there is evidence that the Shangs' used lancing or bloodletting therapeutic practices. Some scholars believe this was a precursor to modern acupuncture, but others strongly differentiate the two.

The Shang dynasty was a shamanistic period in Chinese history. Since many illnesses were thought to be caused by upset ancestors or evil curses, treatment involved consulting an oracle, who would consult "oracle bones." The bones were heated until they cracked, and the pattern of the cracks would reveal the answer to the questions asked to the oracle or shaman.

Therefore, while the Shang dynasty represents the oldest surviving evidence of rudimentary medical practices, it cannot truly be said to be the birth period of what we know today as TCM. The first extant proof of TCM theory comes from the Warring States period (476-221 BC) and the Zhou dynasty (1050-221 BC).

During this period, philosophy and science began to intersect, and the concept of Qi, which forms an essential part of TCM, was developed. This was the start of the movement away from the shamanistic principles of the Shang dynasty to the comprehensive medical system TCM is today.

Following the advent of the Han dynasty (c. 202 BC-220 AD), scholars put together texts that were first written during the Warring States period. This helped the development of TCM.

One of the best-known and most important texts collected during this period is the Yellow Emperor's Inner Canon (Huangdi Nei Jing), sometimes known as the Yellow Emperor's Inner Classic.

Yellow Emperor's Inner Canon

This book is essentially a dialogue between the Yellow Emperor and his physician and ministers. The Yellow Emperor was a legendary Chinese emperor known as Huangdi. He is one of the mythical Three Sovereigns and Five Emperors and is considered a saint in Daoism.

The Yellow Emperor is also credited with introducing various essentials of life to China, including:

- Wood houses

- Boats

- Carts

- Bow and arrow

- Coined money

- A functioning government with institutions

- Silk production (in some stories, it was his wife who introduced this)

The Inner Canon is the first medical book rejecting magic and the spirits as an explanation for illnesses. Rather, it explores concepts like yin yang and wu xing (the Five Phases) linking illnesses. For this reason, it is considered the birth of Traditional Chinese Medicine.

Other classical TCM tomes compiled during the Han dynasty covering the Yellow Emperor's rule and teachings include:

- **Treatise on Cold Damage Disorders and Miscellaneous Illnesses (Shang Han Lun):** This classic combines the practices of yin yang and wu xing, introduced in the Inner Canon, with the first vestiges of drug therapy in China. It covers herbal prescriptions based on mentioned symptoms.

- **Huangdi Bashiyi Nanjing (The Huang Emperor's Canon of Eighty-One Difficult Issues), Known as Nanjing:** The book comprises 81 questions and answers to clarify statements relatively unclear in the Inner Canon. Some concepts examined in the classic include meridians, acupuncture, and diseases.

- **Shennong Ben Cao Jing (Classic of the Materia Medica):** A compilation of Chinese Herbology and medical plants based on oral traditions during the Qin (221-206 BC) and Han dynasties.

The first examples of acupuncture for treating Qi are dated to the Han dynasty (c. 2nd-1st century BC). These indicate that this was the period when TCM was truly born and developed into a comprehensive medical theory.

There have been several developments in Traditional Chinese Medicine since the Han dynasty. One of the most important was the development of inoculation against smallpox in 900-1000 AD. This was the first recorded time that inoculation was used and was a precursor to modern vaccination.

Despite this development, by the 17th century, there was a decline in TCM practices. These practices were considered superstition, and many Chinese people turned to modern, germ-theory-based Western allopathic Medicine. This decline furthered in the 20th century until TCM practices were outlawed in China in 1929.

However, TCM was revived by the Chinese Communist Party in 1949, starting with acupuncture. During the 1950s, interest in TCM continued to grow, and the government promoted this interest during the Cultural Revolution (1966-1976) to ensure China's independence in the field of affordable medical care.

Acupuncture, in particular, became enormously popular in neighboring countries. It was introduced prominently to the West by New York Times (NYT) after James Reston was treated for appendicitis in China in 1971 – a treatment involving acupuncture. Impressed with the results, he published a report in the NYT detailing his experience, resulting in a growing interest in the practice in the West and, in particular, the United States.

The Chinese government has continued to promote TCM in the 20th and 21st centuries, recognizing and understanding its value as a medical and cultural system. In many Chinese hospitals, TCM treatments are integrated with Western medical treatments, making TCM a truly complementary medical practice.

Additionally, many countries, including the United States, have certifications and licenses for TCM providers, especially acupuncturists. A license is a legal requirement for TCM providers to practice in many countries, although it is not the case worldwide.

Understanding Traditional Chinese Medicine Practices

Several beliefs and practices are performed under the banner of TCM, and understanding what each practice entails will help you determine which practice is right for your needs. Some practices include Chinese Herbology, yin and yang, Qigong, acupuncture, acupressure, and wu xing.

Of these, are five TCM branches:

- Qigong, or physical movement

- Acupuncture

- Chinese Dietary Medicine

- Herbology

- Tuina, or massage

Wu Xing

Wu xing, known as the Five Element Theory, the Five Phases, and the Five Agents, is one of the foundational philosophical beliefs of TCM.

In wu xing, five elements make up the material world:

- Wood

- Fire

- Earth

- Metal

- Water

This theory examines how these five elements move and transform and how they are related to each other. In this theory, all parts of the natural world are made of these five elements. These elements are used to categorize natural phenomena according to their elements.

For example, regarding seasons, each season corresponds to an element:

- Wood: spring

- Fire: summer

- Earth: late summer

- Metal: autumn

- Water: winter

Similarly, the elements categorize directions, livestock, fruit, grains, and more. All the items correspond to a certain element and also correspond to each other. For example, wood is related to spring and the east. Therefore, the east also relates to spring.

TCM practitioners use the wu xing theory to explain the relationships between elements of the body, such as body parts, emotions, yin and yang organs, sensory organs, etc. These categorizations form the base for treatment, especially in traditional five-phase acupuncture.

Yin and Yang

Along with wu xing, yin and yang is the key philosophical theory comprising TCM practices. They are key to helping practitioners understand the people's health they are treating and offering diagnoses and treatments.

Yin and yang are opposing yet interconnected forces.

- Yin is the female force. The negative and dark force is represented as the black section of the yin and yang diagram. It represents rest and the right side of the body. However, because it is a "negative" force, it does not mean it is bad – it merely means it is the opposite of yang.

- Yang is the male force. It is the positive, light force represented as the white section of the traditional yin and yang diagram. It represents activity and the left side of the body. Since yin is not a bad force, yang is not a good force – it is merely one of the two essential forces of the universe.

Four Aspects of yin and yang explain the relationship between them:

- They are opposites.

- They are interdependent. There can be no yin without yang, and vice-versa.

- They are mutually transformative. Yin and yang constantly change and transform, but they do so together. If one changes, so does the other. Yin cannot be in flux without yang changing and vice-versa.

- They are mutually consuming. If either yin or yang is out of balance, the other changes, so they reach a new proportion with each other. The interaction of one affects the other, so there is no way for one force to be imbalanced without affecting the other.

TCM holds that yin and yang are normally in balance with each other. When they fall out of balance, they cause a person to fall ill.

For this reason, TCM involves helping a person return to a balanced state of yin and yang energies in the body. All illnesses in TCM fall under one of four categories:

1. Yin in excess

2. Yang in excess

3. A deficient of yin

4. A deficient of yang

In TCM, the effect of yin and yang imbalance is based on Eight Principles.

- Yin Imbalance: Affects the exterior of the body, causes cold, and results in a deficiency of factors in your body that prevent disease

- Yang Imbalance: Affects the interior of the body, causes heat, and results in excess of disease-causing factors in the body

The Five Phases can map how yin and yang change and affect your body. wu xing helps explain the pattern of yin-yang transformation in your body and can be mapped on the organs of your body. The interaction between the elements, wu xing, the interaction between the organs, and how they affect the yin-yang balance is known as Zang-Fu.

The Zang-Fu organs produce the Five Vital Substances essential to life:

- **Qi:** The most basic of the Five Vital Substances, Qi is often considered the building block of the other substances. It is the universal life force that flows through the meridians of a person's body.

- **Blood:** Considered a Yin substance, Blood is the energy that nourishes a person's body and mind. Blood is part of a cycle with Qi – Qi is necessary for the production of Blood, Blood is necessary for the functioning of the Zang-Fu organs, and the Zang-Fu organs are necessary for the production of Qi.

- **Spirit:** The most concentrated form of Yang Qi energy stored in the blood vessels. It is formed through a combination of Qi and Essence and is responsible for thought, understanding, and relating to the people around you. Lack of balance in the amount of Spirit in a person's body results in mental illnesses and trouble with emotional regulation.

- **Essence:** The most concentrated form of Yin Qi energy is stored in the kidneys. It is responsible for the body and soul's growth and development. It flows through the Eight Extraordinary Meridians, is the energy of fertility, and is key in producing semen or menstrual blood.

- **Body Fluids:** Considered Yin substances, Body Fluids are the fluids that lubricate the organs, including tears, spinal fluid, and sweat.

Qigong

Known as Chi Kung, Qigong is essentially a series of exercises designed to help you cultivate your Qi.

However, Qigong is not limited to physical exercise. These exercises include:

- Breathing exercises

- Guided meditation and imagery

- Physical posture exercises

- Qigong exercises can be divided into two parts:

  - Wai Dan: The external elements of Qigong, including physical exercises and mental concentration

  - Nei Dan: The internal elements of Qigong, including guided meditation and visualization

Qigong first involves learning the physical and breathing exercises and coordinating the two. The physical element of Qigong is similar to Tai Chi (but not the same) and is practiced until a person gets every posture down perfectly.

Once the physical element is perfect, practitioners are taught to look for the subtle flow of Qi in the body as they perform physical and breathing exercises. Once they can identify this, the physical part of Qigong is known as moving meditation.

As part of moving meditation, practitioners also practice still meditation. Still, meditation is a series of Qigong postures that are held for longer periods and designed to strengthen your body and increase the flow of Qi in your body.

After practicing moving meditation, practitioners can move on to sitting meditation.

Sitting meditation focuses on breathing and a better understanding of your body and mind function.

Visualization is performed during all three forms of meditation – however, it is not necessary to the process and acts as a Qigong enhancer.

There are three types of Qigong:

- **Medical Qigong:** The practitioner uses Qigong to heal themselves and others.

- **Spiritual Qigong:** The purpose is for the practitioner to reach enlightenment

- **Martial Qigong**: Is used to improve a practitioner's physical capability

TCM generally focuses on medical Qigong. Medical Qigong can be performed by the subject (person looking for healing) using Qigong to heal their Chi imbalance.

Alternatively, the practitioner can also use medical Qigong. Known as Qi Emission, it essentially involves a practitioner emitting Qi from their bodies to bring balance to the patient's Qi, helping to heal them. Generally, Qi Emission is used in self-healing Qi.

Chinese Herbology

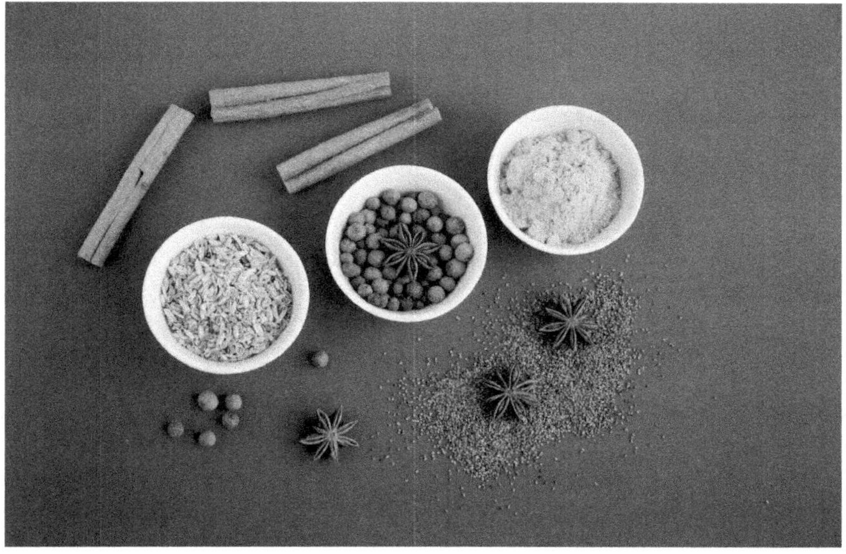

As the name implies, Chinese Herbology uses herbal medications to help balance a person's QI and heal their ailments. Chinese Herbology is not limited to using plant-based elements and medicines; it also uses animal-based ingredients and minerals.

In the past, Chinese Herbology used medicines with ingredients from elements of the human body, such as bones and fingernails. However, most of these medicines are no longer used in modern Herbology practice.

Chinese Herbology uses thousands of ingredients, with over 100,000 medicine recipes depending on a person's ailment. Chinese Herbology medications can be separated into two parts:

- **Chinese Patent Medicine**: This doesn't refer to patents of modern law. Rather, it refers to the formulas because this Chinese Herbology section is standardized.

- **Chinese Herbal Extracts**: As the name implies, this refers to extracts made from herbs converted to powder or granules. These are easier to consume than patent medicine and are significantly easier to make.

Acupuncture and Acupressure

Acupuncture and acupressure focus on regulating the Qi levels in your body.

Acupuncture involves inserting thin, sterile needles into specific points on the body. This practice stimulates your meridians so any Qi imbalance in your body can correct itself.

While acupressure is similar to acupuncture, it does not use needles. Instead, as the name implies, the practitioner applies pressure on a person's skin to reach the same results. While a licensed practitioner should always do acupuncture, it is possible to learn to perform acupressure on yourself.

Since the two are so similar, choosing between them can be challenging. However, as acupuncture involves more training to ensure the practitioner is properly qualified, knows where the pressure points are to insert the needles, and has the skill to ensure the patient feels no pain, acupuncture is often more expensive.

For this reason, people gravitate to acupressure for less serious conditions while opting for acupuncture for more acute conditions. However, this is not a rule; you can choose which practice you feel is right for your needs.

Diet and Lifestyle

In TCM, food fall under five categories:

- Cool natured

- Hot natured

- Cold natured

- Neutral

- Warm natured

The food aims to reach a balance in the body, essentially ensuring your body stays neutral and your Qi stays balanced. Warm and hot-natured foods heat your body, while cool and cold-nature foods cool it.

Ideally, you should balance how much food you consume. Eating too much of one kind can cause an imbalance in your body, resulting in an illness.

Other key elements of a TCM-based diet include:

- Avoiding sweets and deep-fried foods

- Never missing breakfast

- Eating at regulated times

- Consuming proteins with every meal

- Beginning every meal with herbal tea or warm water

You should also tailor your food consumption according to the seasons. For example, increase your warm and hot-natured foods intake in winter, while in the summer, switch to cool and cold-natured foods.

Aside from diet, TCM also concerns a person's lifestyle. Some lifestyle tips followed in TCM include:

- Getting enough sleep and rest, as sleep deprivation can cause illness

- Getting enough daily exercise to boost the circulation of Qi through your body

- Taking positive measures to reduce stress in your life. Some stress reduction methods promoted in TCM include Qigong, Tai Chi, meditation, and deep breathing. You can also take other steps to reduce stress, like practicing Pilates.

- Incorporating acupuncture or acupressure into your lifestyle as a preventative practice and complementary therapy to reduce negative habits like smoking.

- Following a healthy diet recommended by TCM and your TCM practitioner.

- Having a good mental attitude

Chinese Herbal Medicine has evolved over centuries giving us a practical and healthy healing system without the hassle of side effects.

Chapter 2

Diagnosis in Chinese Medicine

Traditional Chinese medicine employs methods for diagnosing human pathological conditions markedly different from typical western diagnoses. Traditional Chinese medicine utilizes herbal products, physical approaches, and psychological techniques to tackle various health issues.

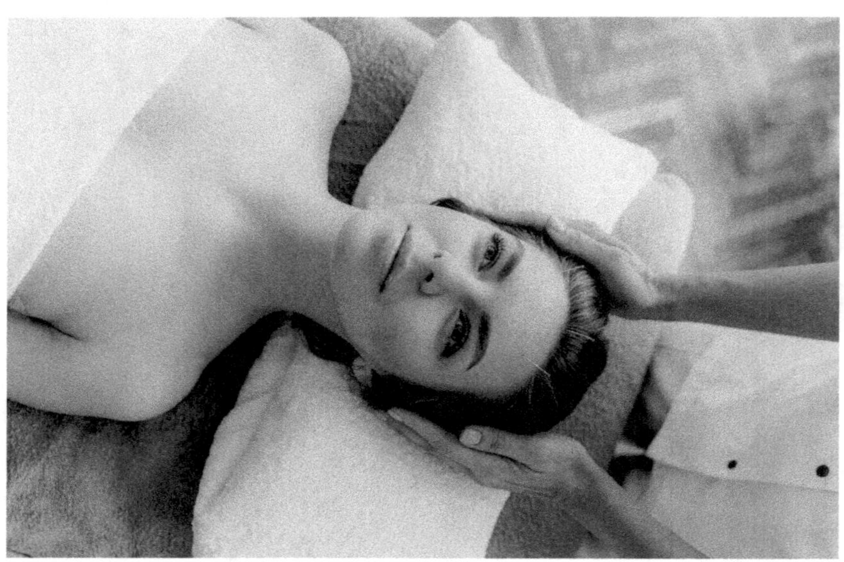

Instead of using stethoscopes, x-ray machines, radiology, and other modern equipment, ancient Chinese medicine specialists have established four main diagnostic methods. Observation, auscultation, olfaction, questioning, and taking the patient's pulse can determine their symptoms. These symptoms are put into a diagnostic syndrome to guide treatment.

These techniques for diagnoses are elaborated upon in the following sections.

Methods of Diagnosis in Chinese Medicine

Inspection (observation), auscultation and olfaction (listening and smelling), interrogation (inquiring or questioning), and palpation are the four most common methods of Chinese medicine diagnosis. How useful each method is, depends on what it does and how it works with other methods to treat health problems.

1. Inspection

Inspection, or observation, is a diagnostic method in Chinese medicine to determine a patient's physical condition before treatment begins. During observation, information about the disease is gathered by looking at how the patient's body and overall appearance have changed.

The Chinese medicine practitioner can tell the patient's symptoms through intentional intuition during the inspection. The patient must be visually examined, and abnormalities found should suggest a diagnosis. Passive association with previous experiences is also significant. A specific symptom can be linked to another, and the diagnosis is made based on other similar inspection experiences.

How Inspection Is Conducted

Inspection is a thorough overall visual examination. The changes in the patient's body shape, appearance, and physical state observed during the inspection are noted. The patient's defense ability, vitals, and clinical symptoms, such as shortness of breath, body color, fatigue, excessive sweat, etc., are also considered in the inspection diagnosis method. The causes of a health problem and its symptoms can be determined by inspecting the patient.

So, a diagnosis is made based on the doctor's knowledge of the patient's symptoms and what the patient can see temporarily.

Tongue Diagnosis

Inspection also includes examining the body and coat of the tongue. The tongue can become quite complicated for patients taking various medications for an extended period or having ongoing health issues. The tongue is examined to determine similarities and differences in tongue evaluations from the tongue's previous stage.

The color, moisture, coating, and vitality of the tongue indicate the state of blood and the quality of body fluids. The shape of the tongue indicates the organ's status, which is the most important factor to consider.

The tip of the tongue represents the lungs and heart; the center represents the spleen and stomach; the sides represent the liver and gallbladder; and the root represents the intestines, urinary bladder, and kidneys.

Normality

A healthy tongue is typically pale red and moist, with a supple body shape that is neither too thin nor too thick. The tongue coat should be white and thin, with a soft and smooth surface free of cracks, and it should move freely.

2. Auscultation and Olfaction

Listening and smelling are referred to as auscultation and olfaction in Chinese medicine. In Chinese herbal medicine, this method of diagnosis entails detecting body odors, listening to the voice, and making breathing sounds.

The abnormal odor and sound emanating from the body could indicate certain issues with the functioning of the internal organs and other previously unnoticed issues. They can also show changes in the organ's yin, yang, and Qi (blood, fluid, and energy).

People who practice Chinese medicine listen to the body for unusual sounds to determine what's wrong, like if an organ isn't working right.

How Auscultation and Olfaction Are Performed

The body is smelled and listened to for abnormalities during this diagnostic method. Sound abnormalities include shortness of breath, frequent crying, sighing, stomach rumbling, moaning, burping, flatulence, and sneezing. The tone of the voice, whether loud or soft, and the joints' clicking are considered.

Odd odors from underarms, urine, body discharge, sweat, stool, and bad breath are examples of odor abnormalities. Generally, rancid "goatish" odors are associated with the liver; rotten or rank odors with the lung; burned odors with the heart; fragrant, cloying, or sweet odors with the spleen; and putrid odors with the kidney.

The strange sounds and smells all have different interpretations for diagnosis. Grinding the teeth while sleeping could indicate a digestive disorder, and clicking of the joints could indicate a lack of circulation and liver yin deficiency. Bad breath could indicate indigestion or a mouth infection. If someone is quiet or won't talk, they usually have a lung, spleen, or kidney problem.

Diagnosing with Listening and Smelling

When using auscultation and olfaction as diagnostic methods in Chinese herbal medicine, certain things are required for accurate diagnosis. Failure to do so could result in misinterpretation and false diagnosis. Some things to remember during your consultation are as follows:

- Wearing perfume is not recommended.

- Don't forget to mention the odor of your secretions and fluids.

- Avoid eating foods with strong odors, such as garlic and chives.

Some body smells and sounds are natural, but auscultation and olfaction will help distinguish what is abnormal from what is not, provide an internal diagnosis and aid in treatment.

3. Interrogation

Interrogation, known as inquiring or questioning, is a common method of getting information from a patient. It is an important examination method because how the patient answers the questions gives important diagnostic signs, reflecting the patient's underlying mental, physical, and emotional conditions. It is the main thing that the Chinese medicine practitioner and the patient will discuss.

Besides, the questioning gives the practitioner a chance to interact with the patient and show their skill and care, which greatly affects how well the therapy works.

Enormous knowledge about the disease and useful information from the patient relating to their condition is required. This method requires time, patience, and active listening because the patient's symptoms must be recognized, and a correct diagnosis must be obtained.

How Interrogation Is Done

The patient is subjected to extensive and thorough questioning to provide diagnostic clues. Some Chinese medicine practitioners follow a standard procedure for questioning patients. First, the patient is quizzed on the integumentary system and the effects of the environment, like cold and heat. The perspiration system for body temperature regulation and the head and body are investigated.

The Chinese medicine practitioner then asks about the patient's bowel evacuation habits and excretory system. The patient's eating habits are investigated next. Concerns about thoracoabdominal disorders and aural comprehension are discussed. The patient will also be asked how often they feel thirsty and how their digestive system works. They are also asked about any previous illnesses or relapses and family illnesses.

Diagnosing with Interrogation

Questions about gynecology and obstetrics are asked of female patients. Questions about andrology will be asked of male patients.

Questions about koplik spots must be asked of children. If the patient is a small child unable to speak or is unconscious, a close relative must answer the questions. Questions should be asked flexibly based on the state of the disease.

The interrogation diagnostic method explains the major characteristics of the disease, its complications, and how it affects the body.

4. Palpation and Pulse Examination

The temperature of the skin, warm or cold; the texture, moist or dry; the surface, raised or flat; and rashes and bruises are all examined during pulse diagnosis. The body is also examined to determine how deep or shallow injuries are and their size and location.

Palpation is the act of feeling with the hands. Palpable areas of the body include the front of the throat and the top of the instep. Using palpation gathers information about the problem and its cause, such as the pain level, numbness, unusual sensations, and lumps. Palpation is approached in two ways in Chinese medicine.

General Palpation

The areas of pain and discomfort are felt in this method. For example, the wrist or ankle for a sprain injury or the abdomen for abdominal pains is felt. In contrast, some Chinese medicine practitioners regularly use the abdominal palpation system for all their patients.

Pulse Taking

This method is the most mysterious of all tests. The radial arteries in both arms' wrists are felt. By applying different amounts of pressure to three areas of the arteries corresponding to three organs in the body, the pathological changes in the bowels and main visceral can be determined.

How Pulse Examination Is Done

The Chinese medicine practitioner places three fingers on the radial artery on the lateral side of the wrist. It must be done on both wrists. There are differences in the depth and force of the pulse in all three fingers; this examination determines the pulse rate.

A taut pulse indicates the body is stressed or has a liver disorder. A deep and slow pulse indicates a lack of energy, Qi deficiency.

Diagnosing with Pulse Examination

When the skin sweats, it can signify that the organs are too hot.

When the skin is dry, the body is thin, the patient is frequently thirsty, and the stool is dry, Yin (moisture) deficiency could be present. Touching your hip and feeling pain on the side of your leg, away from the middle of your body, could signify that your gallbladder channel is blocked.

When the patient's skin is palpated and takes a long time to return medially, has low energy, frequently urinates in the evening, and has lower back pain, it could indicate kidney yang deficiency.

For a more accurate diagnosis from a pulse exam, the patient shouldn't do the following thirty minutes before their appointment:

- Participate in strenuous exercise.

- Consume any hot liquid.

- Overeat

If the patient cannot avoid these prior to the consultation, the pain level must be communicated to the practitioner. Also, the patient must stay calm and comfortable during palpation, so the cause of the disease or body imbalance can be correctly found.

Disharmony in Chinese Medicine

In Chinese medicine, diagnosis is based on a subtle assessment of the patient's disharmony. Each organ system has associations with seasons, food flavors, time of day, emotions, sense organs, etc. These systems work together to keep the body balanced; if one stops working properly, it can throw them off balance.

Patterns of Disharmony

The pattern of disharmony refers to the method of determining the underlying primary disharmony of all clinical manifestations by considering the overall picture of all symptoms and signs.

In Chinese medicine, the pattern represented by the patient's symptoms is not the cause of the disease but rather how the condition manifests. After the pattern is found, the cause imbalance is determined, and a treatment plan is made to bring the body back into balance.

The pattern of disharmony in traditional Chinese medicine can be determined by examining eight major parameters. These are yin and yang, excess and deficiency, internal and external, and hot and cold, and they explain how the seven emotions and pernicious external influences disrupt the body's balance.

They also talk about yin and yang, opposing forces out of balance because of disharmony.

1. The Yin and Yang

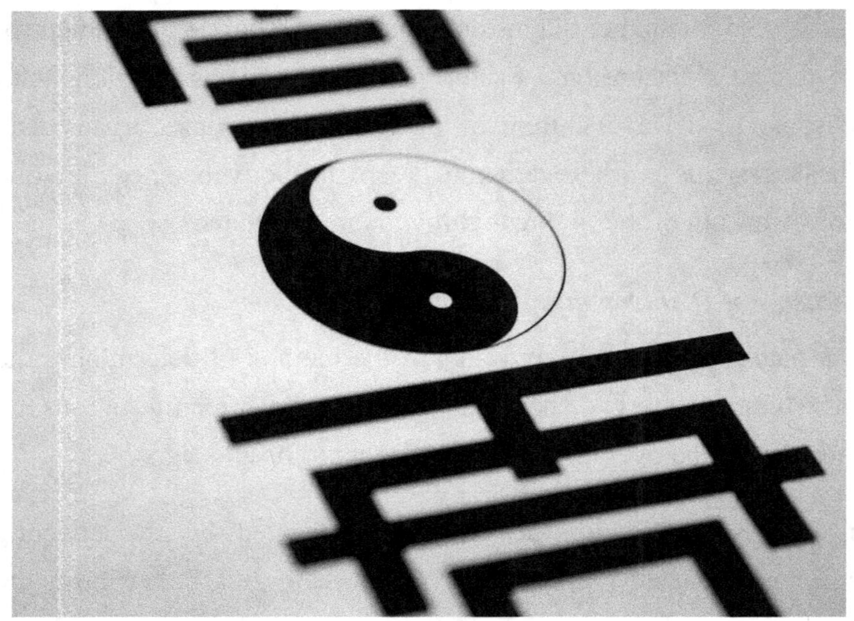

These forces encompass the remaining six basic patterns. The yin represents cold, internal, and deficiency, whereas the yang represents heat, external, and excess. The practitioner looks for signs of yin and yang imbalance on the inside or outside, such as heat or cold, excess or deficiency, and translates them into clinical symptoms to determine where the yin and yang are out of balance.

The Chinese medicine practitioner will diagnose a condition based on the qualities identified during your consultation. For example, if you are cold, slow, and breathing shallowly, the practitioner will diagnose you with cold deficiency yin.

2. Excess and Deficiency

This pattern represents the result of disharmony in the body's resistance to diseases. Weakness, slow movement, organ underperformance, pale face, sweating, shallow breathing, and pain relieved by pressure are symptoms of deficiency. Signs of excess include heavy breathing, forceful movement, and pain that worsens when pressure is applied.

You can help harmonize your body by learning to read it by looking at your medical history, finding excesses and deficiencies in the illnesses you've had, and comparing them to how balance and imbalance are described in Chinese herbal medicine.

3. Internal and External

This pattern indicates the location of the disease. When there is no reaction to a cold, pain in the torso, changes in urine and stool, and chronic disharmony, an internal pattern of disharmony is manifested.

On the other hand, the external pattern of disharmony is abrupt and severe. Some symptoms include a cold, aches all over the body, and fever.

4. Hot and Cold

This pattern reveals the body's activities and the nature of the illness. When someone has a cold, they are slow, sleep in a curled-up position, and are withdrawn. When they are given warmth, their pain is relieved. They prefer warm liquids and have clear, thin body secretions.

In contrast, heat causes rapid body processes, excessive talking, a hot body, a desire for cold beverages, and dark, thick and putrid body secretions.

Pathogenic Factors Related to Chinese Medicine

Pathologies of organ systems, channels, and essential substances are studied to learn what causes disharmony, how it shows, and how it affects the body's balance.

The pathology of essential substances and their disharmonies is as follows:

1. Qi Disharmonies

When Qi works in harmony all over the body, there is wholeness and good health. In contrast, illnesses can arise when Qi is out of balance.

Excess and stagnant qi are related to blockages in the organ systems and channels due to suppressed emotions, poor diet, and traumatic injury. When this is experienced, you feel pain, fullness in the abdomen, and trouble sitting still, and the pain worsens when pressure is applied. When Qi gets blocked, it can get out of balance and cause symptoms like nausea, bloating, and fainting.

Deficient Qi occurs when lack of exercise, bad diet, and respiration problems use up Qi, and it is not replenished. It can cause a weak voice, fatigue, a pale face, and discord in a specific organ system.

2. Shen Disharmonies

Disharmony in Shen is frequently the first sign of developing diseases and other disharmonies. This disharmony is typically caused by imbalance in the seven emotions, accompanied by stagnant Qi and disharmony in the heart system.

Disturbed Shen causes forgetfulness, memory lapses, insomnia, disorganization, and, in extreme cases, madness. Chronic diseases can still be avoided if the Shen (mind) is slightly out of balance.

3. Jing Disharmonies

Jing is a natural part of our being, and we either deplete or replenish it. Sexual problems, birth defects, infertility, and insufficient food are signs of not having enough Jing.

4. Xue Disharmonies

When Xue is deficient throughout the body, the skin becomes dry. It causes blurred vision, hair loss, irregular menstruation, and malnutrition. It is also linked to emotional stress, Qi depletion, and blood loss.

Excess or stagnant Xue is associated with direct tissue damage, such as falling from an elevated surface. Sharp, stabbing pain and swollen organs are among the symptoms.

5. Jin-Ye Disharmonies

Dry eyes, hair, lips, and skin are symptoms of Jin-Ye deficiency. Excess Jin-Ye is associated with swelling, fluid accumulation, and edema.

Only during pregnancy is an increase in Xue and Jin-Ye, a normal part of how the body works and is not always a sign of too much disharmony.

In traditional Chinese medicine, organs and their patterns of disharmony are listed below.

Heart System

The heart's primary function is to pump blood. In traditional Chinese medicine, the heart is where the mind lives. Due to this, it is significant in sleep patterns and psychological and mental disorders.

Heart system disharmony is shown by too much laughing and crying, trouble falling asleep, agitation, poor memory, heart failure, irregular pulse, purple lips, a slow heartbeat, and chest pain.

Lung System

In traditional Chinese medicine, the lungs control the immune system, controlling breathing and sweating. Coughs, asthma, allergies, dry skin, low energy, lack of sweating, sore throat, and long periods of grief are symptoms of general lung disharmony.

Kidney System

When we run out of energy from the spleen and lungs, the kidney acts as a body reservoir. In traditional Chinese medicine, the kidney is associated with growth and reproduction, not only urination. Besides the natural loss of energy that comes with aging, this degeneration is also caused by poor diet and lifestyle choices.

Lack of exercise, hearing loss, impotence, bed-wetting, premature aging, and retarded growth are symptoms of kidney disharmony.

Spleen System

In Chinese herbal medicine, this is the major digestive organ through which we obtain Qi from the food we eat and the air we breathe. The spleen is also the site of blood formation. Its job is to get nutrients from our food, make the energy we need every day, keep the blood in its vessels, and keep the organs in place.

Internal spleen problems can cause weakness, loss of appetite, malnutrition, chronic diseases, bloody stools, heavy periods, and pain and fullness in the abdomen.

Comparison between Western Diagnosis and Chinese Diagnosis

Western medicine uses lab tests to diagnose patients and focuses on symptom elimination rather than addressing the underlying causes of illness. On the other hand, Chinese medicine focuses on the body's overall response to treatment while acknowledging the body as an interconnected system. In Western diagnosis, the cause of a patient's illness is found by looking at each symptom individually. However, in Chinese diagnosis, the pattern of disharmony looks at all symptoms simultaneously.

Western medicine employs pharmaceutical therapies and prescribes specific drugs for disease treatment. They recommend surgery, physical therapy, and pharmaceuticals based on objective descriptions of the disease.

On the contrary, in Chinese medicine, the person is treated comprehensively—mind, body, soul, and spirit—rather than just their symptoms. The patient's symptoms are gathered through subjective thinking, questioning, palpation, listening, smelling, and observation. These symptoms are put into the diagnostic syndrome mentioned earlier.

Patients with chronic functional problems, particularly those in Western medicine, who cannot determine the cause, but have unpleasant symptoms, could benefit from Chinese medicine treatment.

Chapter 3

Philosophies behind Chinese Medicine

The first few chapters of this book uncovered the unique history behind traditional Chinese medicine and how it eventually broke through the mainstream, overcoming thousands of years of bias and ignorance. As previously established, traditional Chinese medicine is an intricate study that takes a holistic view of the human body and has not changed much since its inception. The driving concept behind the practice is referred to as Qi or the vital force of life that surges through the body. Understanding this philosophy is integral to gaining a sense of the key pillars of Chinese medicine. A few more concepts branch off from there. Any imbalance in the Qi leads to disease and illness, and the complementary life forces that work in tandem, yin, and yang, are equally important.

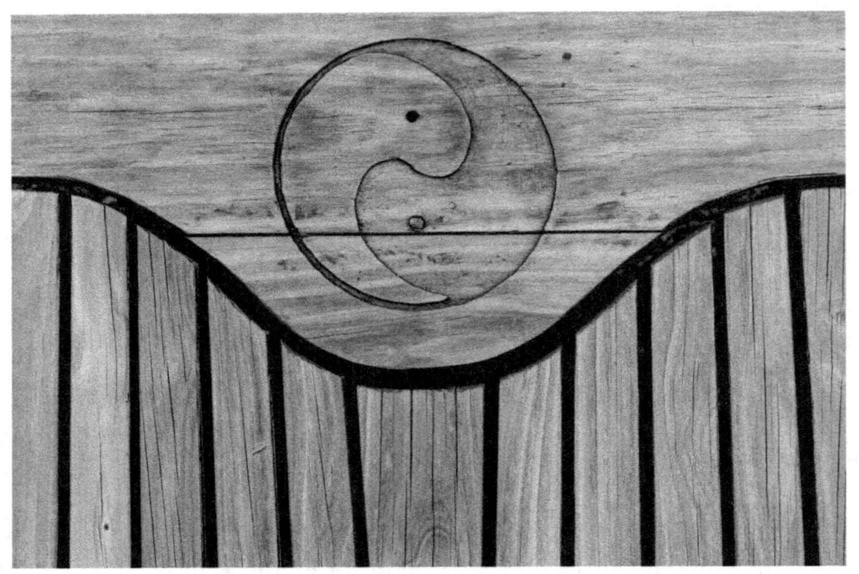

While aspects of traditional Chinese medicine are rather complicated and require years of study to implement effectively, some key precepts can be made more accessible to the layman. This chapter will help elucidate the central philosophies and grant a better understanding of how they affect the practice of Chinese medicine.

What Is Qi?

If you've ever tried an acupuncture session and talked about Chinese herbs, you probably heard quite a bit about Qi from your acupuncturist. Or, they might have referred to it as Chi, which is essentially the same word – although the latter indicates a truer pronunciation in Chinese. As mentioned earlier, Qi is the vital life force that surges throughout your body. Therefore, you must be mindful of the air, water, and food you consume to keep the Qi nourished. In a more substantial version of the philosophy, some traditional Chinese medicine practitioners take into account the vital fluids and energy that flows through their bodies.

So, in many ways, Qi is exceptionally concerned with what we take into our bodies, creating parts of us and our ecosystem. However, another part of the philosophy focuses on what has already become part of our being and is released to continue life's cycle. Any imbalances in this cycle or interruptions in the flow of life force will cause a plethora of human ailments, from the mental, physical and emotional.

It's worth mentioning that this concept of a central life-giving force that courses through our bodies is not singular to Chinese culture. Most cultures have a variation of this idea, from the Ancient Egyptians to the Prana in India and the force known as Ki in Japan. Native Americans also refer to the life force as The Great Spirit. The main difference is that this concept is applied to the practice of medicine, and tremendous weight is placed on the life force that must move with ease and be in perfect alignment to maintain good health.

Of course, the Qi comprises other "mini" systems coursing throughout the body, one of which is heavily informed by the philosophy of yin and yang. To go back again to the situational example of a visit to the acupuncturist, you probably have a vague idea that they would immediately try their best to balance the Qi, working with other branches of the philosophies that make up the backbone of the practice - the meridians (explained later). The basic principle to glean is that the Qi is the starting point for most of the intellectual underpinnings of Traditional Chinese Medicine.

Therefore, the primary aim of Traditional Chinese Medicine is to optimize health and well-being by cultivating a smooth, powerful, and balanced flow of Qi throughout the body. It is believed that any blockage in the body's life force can be alleviated through a combination of tai chi, acupuncture, herbs, and many medicinal practices that have been employed for thousands of years.

The Yin and Yang

For Gen-Xers and older Millennials reading this book, everyone will probably remember the obsession with yin and yang fashion accessories in the 1990s. From chokers to t-shirts, tote bags, etc., the yin and yang symbol was plastered on countless items throughout that period. It was a nod to New Age-y spirituality that became more popular in the West, although the symbol was divorced from its original meaning. Of course, this blatant commercial appropriation of an important symbol represents one of the less savory aspects of the 1990s, which people tend to gloss over for nostalgic reasons. Many people don't necessarily know its meaning or understand the importance of yin and yang in Chinese medicine. This is a shame since there is no real way of understanding Traditional Chinese Medicine or Qi without understanding the concept of yin and yang.

In essence, yin is the portion of the Qi that is cold, passive, heavy, and even dark. It represents the more physical or brutal part of the universe. By contrast, the yang is nebulous, dry, and rather aggressive. So, quite different from the watered-down "good versus evil" spiel we are used to hearing from pop culture, the concept of yin and yang is rather complicated and a bit more involved.

The yin and yang do not exist without one another and are considered complementary forces. They must be kept in proper balance for the Qi to flow throughout the body at a normal pace without being over-activated or blocked. When the yin and yang are properly balanced, they are well-defined and can imbue the individual with good health and balanced emotions and create an overall sense of well-being.

Regarding its applicability in Chinese medicine, the yin is associated with the lower body parts, while the yang is associated with the upper body and back. Considering their interconnectivity, it means diseases in traditional Chinese medicine cannot be treated separately. Both are interdependent forces, and only their harmonious coexistence leads to good health.

It does not mean the yin and yang can only be static forces to achieve good health. They are in constant flux, which is necessary. What causes problems is a lack of balance, leading to illness. For example, when the yin leaves your body feeling cold, there is an excess of that particular force, creating illnesses like insomnia and dry mouth. On the other hand, when there is a deficiency in the yang, you suffer from cold limbs and a sickly complexion. So, good health is maintained when there is a balance between the yin and yang and how it interacts with wu xing (explained later) and the body's overall Qi.

The Meridians

If the Qi is the overriding life force charging throughout your body, and the yin and yang are the different elements of that force maintaining a balance, what are the pathways to achieve this? This concept is called the meridians, or the channels the Qi uses to move through the body. This philosophy is used to pinpoint the energy vessels in the body that help maintain a good balance. The meridians are well organized and follow clear pathways, which traditional Chinese medicine practitioners know how to pinpoint. They function as an interconnected network that looks akin to an underground railway system - hardworking, high functioning, with many interconnected paths linking them to one another and maintaining the same goal of keeping the body in excellent shape. These energy vessels are crucial to acupuncture, and the acupuncturists maintain their equilibrium, keeping the pathways free and fully functioning pathways equilibrium. The concept of the meridians is similar to a circulatory and nervous system in Western medicine, except it's not a physical entity exactly.

There are twelve primary meridians commonly referred to as the principal meridians, and these are divided into the yin and yang groups in different parts of the body. The yin meridian's central energy vessel emanates from the arm and moves through the lung, heart, and pericardium. The yang meridians of the arm are the large intestine, small intestine, and triple burner. The yin meridian of the leg is the spleen, kidney, and liver. The yang meridians of the leg are the stomach, bladder, and gallbladder.

In addition to the twelve standard meridians, the eight extraordinary vessels connect to these different pathways flowing through the body. They are responsible for the connecting wei - the defensive part of the body's Qi - and the yuan - the parental part of the Qi. Acupuncture is one form of Chinese medicine that connects these different pathways, clearing any "traffic jams" so things move clearly and efficiently within the body.

Wu Xing

Another pillar of Traditional Chinese Medicine is wu xing, which refers to the five elements of nature representing movement or change. This theory is central to the medicinal practice and cannot be divorced from achieving a holistic understanding of Qi. Wu xing charts elements that constantly move between yin and yang, such as wood, fire, earth, metal, and water.

This theory of the five elements is derived from the ancient Chinese diligently observing the evolving patterns of nature around them. "Wu" is Chinese for five, and "xing" is translated to the elements, although it can also mean phases, transformations, or forces, depending on the context. These descriptions of the five elements are not static and can also describe the dynamic interactions occurring within the body and nature. Each element can describe a phase of constant movement and is used to maintain a relative balance with the rest of the elements. In summary, the elements represent how the movements of Qi are guided throughout the body. Contained within are all the basic materials and movements that are found in the universe. All the body's internal organs are associated with the five elements. The following is more information on each:

Wood

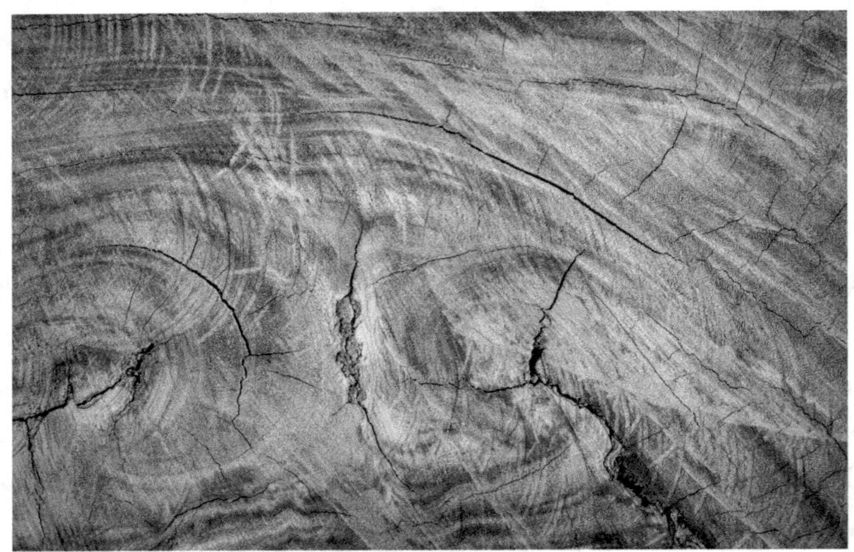

This element describes a period of flourishing and growth. It represents spring and a rejuvenated sense of life, bringing an indelible sense of vitality. This element energy is seen to be moving outwards instead of inwards. So, wood represents growth in all its manifestations and is often associated with periods of childhood and adolescence.

Fire

The next element is fire, which represents summer, filled with warmth and activity. In this sense, fire is filled with energetic movement and is considered an upward ascending force. It signifies a feeling of connection and productivity in work, the emotionality behind making familial decisions, maintaining social networks, etc. Fire is seen as entirely positive and not negative, as it sometimes is in other practices.

Earth

Earth is associated with balance but does not relate directly to one of the four yin and yang movements. It is a stable centralizing force that metaphorically signals that the fruits of labor are ripe for the picking. Since it represents the changes between seasons, traditional Chinese medicine often sees it as the axis around which other phases orbit. If the previous elements are to be treated solely as phases, then the earth phase is the one from which we reap the benefits of the fire phase, settling comfortably into our lives and watching our families grow.

Metal

Metal represents the substance and the transformational phase - from which yang energies emerge and is really connected to the yin. It represents the cleansing reset offered by autumn when energy moves inwards. The energy we produce is internalized, and we try to reduce our stressors in response to achieve balance. The metal element is poignant in many ways since it means we are drawing from hard-earned wisdom won through evolving and learning, and it is representative of the need to devote our energies to becoming more mindful of the passage of time.

Water

The final phase is water, which signifies winter when all energy forces move downwards to achieve a sense of calm. Hence, things become colder and more insular. It is synonymous with this idea of rest and preparing for moving energies upward once again. It is where the yin is found, and a new cycle can begin.

Winter also has negative connotations, but this is not the case in traditional Chinese medicine. None of the elements possess qualities that should make you wary of them. Since they are all treated as essential transformational phases, they have neutral connotations, and the extent to which you should extrapolate different meanings or over-interpret them through a purely cultural lens does not work in the context of medicine.

So, how do these phases work together? The elements support and feed into each other. The extent they can move harmoniously together is reflected in the changing seasons in the world and, by extension, how that rejuvenating force is translated within the body. In therapeutic terms, traditional Chinese medicine practitioners note that it is vital that the elements nourish one another and that the movements are circular: things cannot happen out of order for the body if we want it to function well. The practice of Chinese medicine ultimately comes down to ensuring the phases cycle healthily throughout the body; if there is an excess of one element, it disrupts the much sought-after balance. Therefore, steadily keeping things flowing where they need to is the whole point of the practice.

Western Medicine and Traditional Chinese Medicine

As you might have guessed, there are quite a few differences between the practices of Western medicine and traditional Chinese medicine. Of course, the ultimate outcome or intention is shared - to get well and be healthy. However, their histories and how they were developed are entirely different.

The development of Western medicine is predicated on hypotheticals and deductions. Eastern medicine follows a more inductive approach. Furthermore, Western medicinal practices have always had a clear delineation between health and disease, whereas traditional Chinese medicine looks to have a balanced state versus an unbalanced one. You don't have to wait till you're seriously ill to reap the benefits of traditional Chinese medicine.

A few years ago, there was a notion that you had to choose between the two practices, and your health depended upon not being suckered into something that felt new age-y without many scientific studies. Thankfully, these binaries have long disappeared, and so has the stigma surrounding much of traditional Chinese medicine, which is known to have well-documented benefits. For example, people are encouraged to see a fertility specialist if they're trying to conceive while also taking Chinese herbs and having countless acupuncture sessions to achieve desirable results. Both approaches, while distinct, have plenty of value.

The philosophies in traditional Chinese medicine, informing the ideas behind wu xing, qi, the meridians, and the five elements, are crucial to understanding its central approach: a desire to achieve balance in the body. Harnessing the power of Qi and letting that life force or energy flow without impediments is vital to achieving a sense of well-being. Practitioners understand that most problems arise when the Qi is blocked or the meridians aren't allowing the energy force to move unimpeded throughout the body. Chinese medicine practitioners aim to restore flow and balance, and all treatment is prescribed with that in mind.

The most effective methods to correct imbalances in the body are diet therapy, massage, herbal medicine, Chinese exercises, meditation, and acupuncture. Some practitioners recommend that people follow all these regimens' elements as part of their daily routines, with the idea that they can work together to achieve balance. Others encourage certain parts of these practices more than others to treat only specific ailments. It is really up to the professional and the issues the patient wants to solve.

On the other hand, Western medicine focuses primarily on pharmaceutical therapies to help address health issues. Furthermore, while a general practitioner might recommend basic dictums like maintaining a healthy diet and exercise, they don't usually tell patients to embark on major programs as preventive measures, which is part of the course for as traditional Chinese medicine. However, Western doctors have recognized that practices burnished for thousands of years by their Eastern colleagues have tremendous value and can be life-changing for many of their patients. So much so that taking Chinese herbs while visiting your oncologist for tests is not unheard of and comes highly recommended these days. Also, health insurance companies are more willing to cover acupuncture in many states, which is a boon to everyone wanting to maintain good health and balance between visits to the general practitioner.

Traditional Chinese medicine is a complicated study with different philosophies that practitioners devote many years to master.

Traditional Chinese medicine, in most of its forms, is easily accessible in most regions. Your health and balanced Qi are just an appointment away from being revitalized. However, before visiting the first traditional Chinese medicine practitioner you come across, researching their credentials (even if friends and family have referred them) is advisable. Many inexperienced practitioners and con artists exist, and you will suffer the consequences concerning your health and finances. With an accredited practitioner, your life will undoubtedly change for the better.

Chapter 4

Cupping and Gua Sha

In traditional Chinese medicine, Qi (energy) drives the body. Its imbalance inhibits the Qi from flowing freely, resulting in pain, inflammation, and several other ailments. This disruption of Qi and the development of health-related issues cause blood stagnation or blood stasis. Gua Sha and cupping are centuries-old techniques used in traditional Chinese medicine to promote blood flow, reduce inflammation and pain, and slow down chronic disease developments. These techniques unblock the Qi and promote its free flow in the body. Both methods are based on the same principle, with slight variations in the process and the tools used.

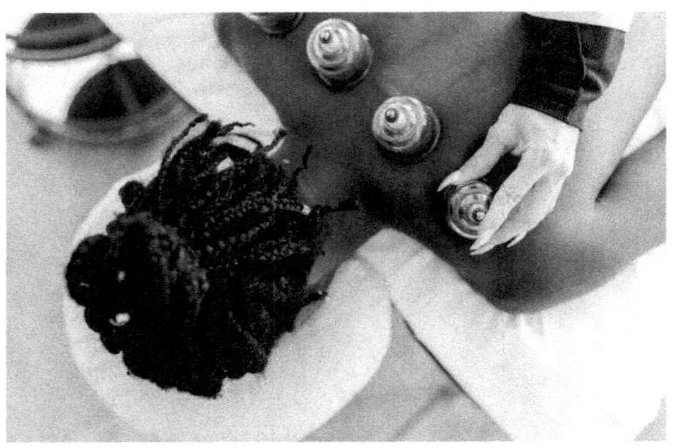

This chapter teaches about cupping and Gua Sha, their uses, the therapy process, related side effects, and much more. The first half of the chapter provides extensive details about the cupping technique, and the other half explains Gua Sha.

What Is Cupping?

It's a technique used in traditional Chinese medicine that involves applying suction cups on the skin. The application creates a vacuum, allowing the cups to stick firmly. The suction created through the cups at different body areas breaks blood stagnation. Suction cups in this technique are made with glass, silicone, or plastic for virtually any skin type.

The cupping technique stimulates blood and lymphatic flow to provide nutrients, remove toxins, and facilitate healing. The improved blood flow after cupping promotes general health and balance, relieves pain, and effectively treats several medical conditions. Once applied, the cups can be left in specific areas or maneuvered by using a lubricant to slide the cups elsewhere. The treatment leaves perfect round marks, which are painless and disappear in a few days.

Types of Cupping Therapies

There are two main cupping techniques called wet and dry cupping. In wet cupping, the skin is pierced with a fine needle. The suction cups on the top limit the amount of blood coming out. On the other hand, dry cupping doesn't involve cutting or piercing the skin.

These two cupping methods are the basis of several cupping practices mentioned below.

Massage Cupping

After placing suction cups on the body, the therapist maneuvers and slides the cups over the skin, replicating the experience of a massage.

Needle Cupping

This practice is a fusion of acupuncture and cupping. Acupuncture needles are applied over the skin first, followed by placing suction cups to conceal the needles within.

Facial Cupping

Suction cups made of silicone are used on the face to detoxify and rejuvenate the skin.

Water Cupping

Around one-third of each suction cup is filled with lukewarm water and inverted to produce a vacuum and the desired effects.

During the cupping session, your therapist will ignite alcohol, paper, or dry herbs in the suction cup to create a vacuum, effectively pulling out defective blood and toxins.

The Process of Cupping

Cupping varies depending on the treatment required. A therapist conducts the procedure with the patient lying on a table, face down, or up. The position is determined by the area requiring treatment. In dry cupping, the practitioner ignites herbs, alcohol, or paper placed in suction cups. As soon as the flames extinguish, the cups are immediately placed on the affected areas of the body.

Burning these materials inside suction cups creates a vacuum when placed on the skin. The vacuum lifts the skin within the cup. Glass suction cups use this method of burning flammable materials for suction. The same effect is achieved using modern-day suction cups, including pumps to remove air from the cup, allowing the practitioner to control the suction according to the therapy's requirements. The cups can be left in a specific area or moved around by stretching their cups.

Wet cupping uses the same procedure as dry cupping. The only difference is that the areas of skin are pierced with needles or cut to release toxins and a small amount of blood from the body. The suction cups are placed on the skin and left for 3 minutes. The cups are removed, and a needle piercing or cut is made to draw out toxins and blood. In some cases, pressure is applied for several minutes to speed up blood flow before placing the cups for the second time.

Whether dry or wet cupping, both methods are not painful but result in discomfort. In a typical cupping session, 3 to 5 cups are placed in specific areas for effective treatment. The number of suction cups can increase depending on the condition. You can expect the skin to develop red, circular bumps that go away within two weeks.

Although the cupping method doesn't involve the direct use of herbs, the process of Moxibustion or moxa is used alongside cupping. In Moxibustion or moxa, medicinal herbs are burned near the skin for a warming therapeutic effect. The cupping practitioner might also add herbal medicine in conjunction with moxa for improved outcomes in diseases like asthma.

Uses and Benefits of Cupping

The cupping technique treats an array of medical conditions. Here's a brief overview.

Reduces Pain and Inflammation

Injuries of the musculoskeletal system, pain, and inflammation can be effectively controlled and healed through cupping. The technique helps reduce pain and inflammation by increasing the blood flow to these areas.

Release of Toxins

The blood flow created through cupping helps the body reduce toxins using the lymphatic system. This increased blood flow triggers tissues to release the trapped toxins naturally.

Reduces Anxiety

Cupping stimulates the parasympathetic nervous system. When activated, the system slows down the heart rate, improves digestion, and triggers a chemical release to manage the hormonal imbalance.

Treating Congestion and Asthma

Congestion occurs due to bronchitis, asthma, and the common cold. The suction of the cups breaks the phlegm, relieving congestion. This method increases blood and oxygen flow to the lungs, improving respiration.

Colon Blockage

When the parasympathetic system activates, digestion improves as more blood is pumped to the digestive tract, increasing peristalsis.

Besides being a traditional treatment in traditional Chinese medicine, the technique's effectiveness is recognized and used in several health-related disciplines like sports medicine. Muscle injuries, strains, and stiff joints are common sports injuries treated using cupping and Gua Sha techniques.

Mitigating Spasms

Spasms commonly occur due to excessive strain on the muscles, making them contract involuntarily. During a spasm, the muscle fails to relax, resulting in severe pain and inflammation. These spasms also limit the flow of blood and nutrients to vital organs like the brain. Cupping prevents cramps by targeting the affected muscles. They increase circulation, resolving the issue within no time.

Here's a list of several medical; conditions that can be treated with cupping.

- Preventing the incidence and controlling symptoms of autoimmune diseases.

- Effective in controlling symptoms of arthritis, fibromyalgia, and carpal tunnel syndrome.

- Improves the function of internal organs like the heart, stomach, and lungs.

- Several other conditions include:

- Chronic obstructive pulmonary disease (COPD).

- Acne, shingles, varicose veins, stretch marks, wrinkles, and other skin-related conditions.

- Facial paralysis.

- Cough and dyspnea.

- Hypertension.

- Asthma and congestion.

An array of other medical and health-related issues are treated with cupping. It's essential to dedicate time to research your problem and find the right approach when attempting cupping yourself. Still, visiting a certified cupping practitioner will make your job much easier as they have the expertise to identify your medical condition, introduce you to the best method, and guide you through the process.

Side Effects of Cupping

The side effects associated with cupping include circular marks, discoloration, and dizziness. Also, there are chances of scarring and hematoma formation on the cupping site. The cupping technique is avoided in several conditions like burns, wounds, blood thinning, and trauma. The skin you choose for cupping should not have veins, arteries, or nerves beneath. Furthermore, areas like body orifices, lymph nodes, and eyes cannot be cupped.

What Is Gua Sha?

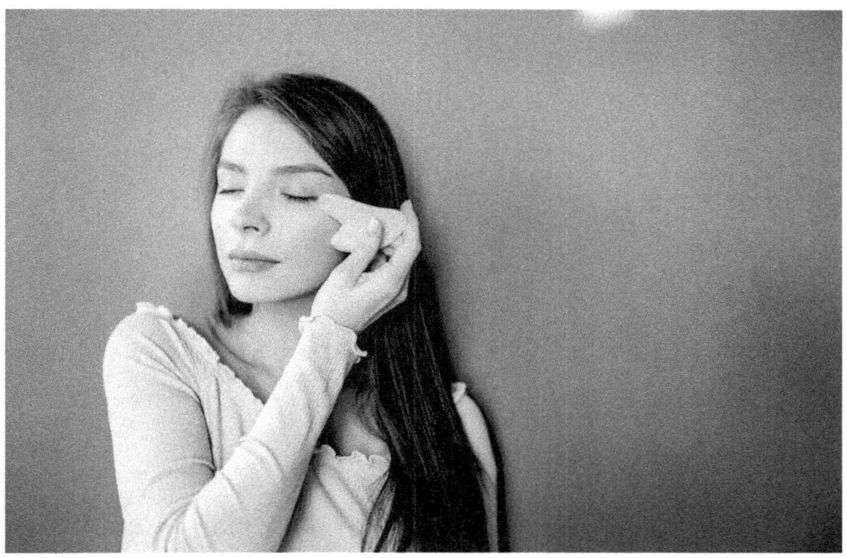

As explained earlier, the basis for cupping and Gua Sha are the same. Both aim at promoting the movement of Qi (energy) throughout the body. According to TCM, the blockage of Qi results in stiffness, pain, and diseases. While cupping involves using suction cups, Gua Sha uses a specialized tool to rub against the skin with pressure. This method helps break down tissues, improves joint mobility, and increases blood and lymph flow to the treated area. Gua Sha results in light bruising that appears as red or purple spots. While the Gua Sha technique seems easier than cupping, both techniques require a certain level of knowledge and practice to develop expertise.

Types of Gua Sha Techniques and Tools

For an effective Gua Sha therapy, selecting the appropriate Gua Sha tool and stone is crucial. Each device has different characteristics, shapes, and sizes, making them suitable for specific areas of the body and for treating certain issues. Traditional Chinese medicine professionals believe in the effects of stones on the body. Each stone makes the tool possesses different characteristics according to the treatment. Here are the materials and tools required for various Gua Sha therapies.

Types of Tools

S-shaped tools can be easily used on the hands, feet, shoulders, neck, and back. The device is available in several materials and is a good choice for beginners practicing Gua Sha.

The fin tool is designed like a fin with three sides for scrapping. The wide shape allows the practitioner to apply the required pressure and is ideal on the biceps, triceps, shoulders, legs, and thighs.

Dolphin-shaped tool provides a firm grip and is an excellent choice for deep massage. Areas of the body with fat or deep muscles like the thighs and glutes require this tool for Gua Sha. Smaller versions of these tools are also available for facial use.

The spoon tool provides easy control and facilitates the practitioner to adjust pressure with simple maneuvers. The tool releases muscle tension by activating acupressure points.

Several other shapes, like the crescent, long bar, and wave, are also quite popular among Gua Sha practitioners. Now that we have covered a basic overview of Gua Sha tool shapes, let's dig into the different materials these tools are made of.

Jade

Jade is a widely used stone in Gua Sha, prevalent in traditional Chinese medicine for its cooling effect and the ability to balance the body's energy. Other benefits of using jade include improvement in digestion and reducing stress build-up.

Rose Quartz

According to traditional Chinese medicine, rose quartz represents love, healing, and compassion. The stone has calming properties and can be used on sensitive skin. Besides reducing wrinkles and acne, rose quartz can drain toxins and negative energy from the body.

Bian Stone

Like rose quartz, the Bian stone has been used for its healing properties since ancient times. The stone users claim it has blood pressure regulation abilities, making it an ideal material for complete body Gua Sha therapies.

Clear Quartz

It's one of the rarest materials and is called the master healer. The stone is believed to improve clarity and calm while balancing the mind, spirit, and body. It's a great choice for treating various skin conditions and is compatible with every skin type.

Amethyst

It's a striking purple-colored stone you might have seen used in jewelry. Amethyst is regarded for its stress-reducing properties and leaves a cooling effect on the skin. The stone is claimed to have antibacterial properties, making it a feasible choice for infectious skin conditions.

The Process of Gua Sha

Depending on the issue and the area requiring treatment, an appropriate Gua Sha tool is selected. Several variations of Gua Sha are mentioned below.

Traditional Gua Sha

This traditional method is widely used in TCM. The practitioner uses smooth-edged Gua Sha tools to scrape the skin. This method aims to improve blood and Qi circulation, reduce inflammation, and decrease stiffness in muscles and joints.

Facial Gua Sha

It's the most popular method and has skyrocketed over the past few years due to its positive results. This method reduces puffiness and facial inflammation, relieves tension, and lowers sinus pressure.

Graston Technique

This technique is similar to the traditional Gua Sha and targets tendons, fascia, and deep muscles rather than focusing on the skin and capillaries. The Graston technique is specifically used to promote collagen production and inhibit pain.

Gua Sha's movements must be smooth, gentle, and always in one direction. The movements and the specialized Gua Sha tools require the proper knowledge and a certain level of training.

Gua sha and cupping are primarily massage techniques with proven benefits for various medical conditions. Like cupping, no specific medicinal herbs are used when practicing the Gua Sha technique. Depending on your ailment, the practitioner might add acupuncture or herbal medicine to control the symptoms or address the root cause of the issue.

Uses and Benefits of Gua Sha

Besides a facial skin rejuvenating technique, Gua Sha treats several diseases and medical conditions.

Reducing Muscle Pain

Gua Sha techniques reduce stiff muscles and joints by increasing the blood flow to these areas. A single session of Gua Sha can significantly reduce the pain, whether neck or chronic back pain.

Controlling Chronic Conditions

Several medical conditions need life-long management and compliance to prevent their progress. Diabetic neuropathy is a condition that develops in patients with poor blood sugar control. These high glucose levels damage nerves and affect the function of virtually every organ. Gua Sha on the legs and feet of chronic diabetic patients aids in controlling blood sugar levels and preventing nerve damage.

Mitigating Perimenopause Discomfort

Perimenopause is the transition period after a woman enters menopause causes mood changes, hot flashes, and sleep problems. Gua Sha sessions for perimenopausal women can reduce these symptoms, making coping through the transition period easier.

Here's a list of several other conditions Gua Sha techniques claim to treat.

- Carpal tunnel syndrome

- Boosts immune system.

- Reduces the incidence of cold and fever.

- Tendon rupture.

- Joint stiffness.

Side Effects of Gua Sha

There are no evident side effects or risks associated with Gua Sha. However, these techniques might not be suitable for individuals with the following:

- A medical condition involving veins.

- Thin blood (people who take blood thinning meds)

- Deep vein thrombosis.

- Superficial wound, ulcer, or a skin infection involving the complete body.

While Gua Sha and cupping have an array of benefits and uses in traditional Chinese medicine, the healthcare industry today is still unable to identify the effectiveness of these techniques due to a lack of research. Still, the study reveals their efficacy in improving blood circulation, reducing inflammation and joint stiffness, and protecting internal organs. When choosing between cupping and Gua Sha, most individuals get confused as both techniques ultimately aim at alleviating Qi stagnation.

Both methods are proven effective in providing short-term relief for chronic pain and inflammation and controlling the symptoms of a long list of medical conditions. Further research is being carried out to explore and recognize the possible benefits of these ancient techniques. Most people prefer a certified practitioner, but some opt to perform these techniques themselves. If you want to perform these techniques yourself, it is recommended to dedicate time to research. Start by understanding why you need the treatment.

After identifying the cause, study different cupping and Gua Sha techniques to know which will suit you best. Lastly, ensure you understand the technique and the step-by-step process before you begin. A few therapy sessions are an excellent idea before practicing these techniques. Furthermore, opt for training sessions by a certified practitioner to thoroughly understand the method, its uses, benefits, and much more.

Chapter 5

Moxibustion

Based on traditional Chinese medicine, Moxibustion is an external treatment that entails burning mugwort leaves. This herb burned close to the skin's surface with a heating stick, enhances healing when used in conjunction with acupuncture. When the mugwort is burned, it produces a sweet fragrant smoke absorbed through the skin. The heat from the burning herb stimulates circulation, enhancing the healing of muscles, tendons, and ligaments. For more than 2,500 years, Moxibustion has been used to dredge meridians and regulate Qi in the blood. This treatment can be used preventatively and therapeutically to cure diseases like colds or flu.

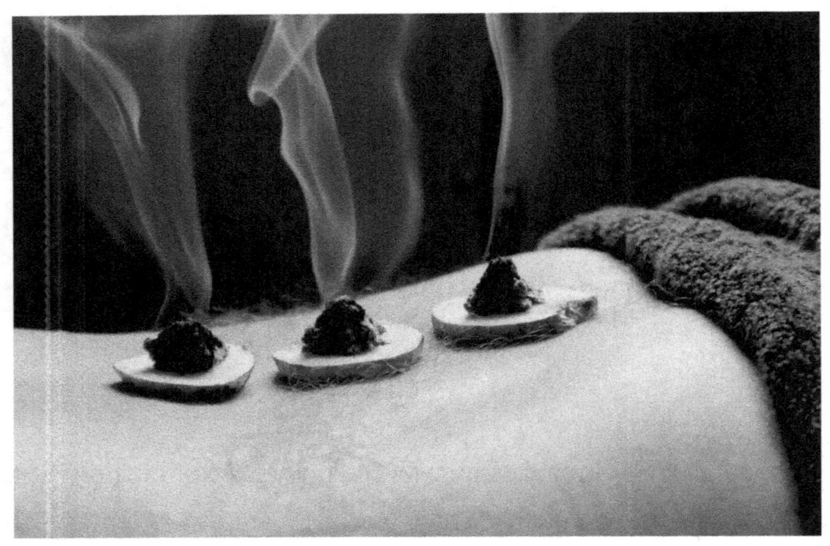

A Brief History of Moxibustion and Its Development

Chinese medical texts from the pre-Qin dynasty, including Zuo Zhuan—which records a discussion about a disease that occurred in 581 B.C.—are considered the earliest written records of Moxibustion. The Mawangdui Silk Books, found in a tomb dating from the Han dynasty (around 168 B.C.), document using Moxibustion to treat medically advanced diseases such as arrhythmia and swelling caused by clots. The Inner Canon of Huangdi contains many Moxibustion treatments implying that Moxibustion origin is closely related to diseased characteristics and living habits of the northern Alpine nation in Su wen, Yi fa fang Yi Lun.

Moxibustion has a wide array of applications in traditional Chinese medicine. A study published from 1954–2007 showed that more than 300 different diseases were treated with Moxa at some point during the research. Some treatable diseases included fatigue, chronic back pain, and aging-related problems. Moxibustion can be classified into the following:

- Traditional Moxibustion: The burning of a specially prepared herb

- Drug Moxibustion: Burning dried mugwort leaves or preparations

- Modern Moxa Therapy: Using electrical devices instead of herbs to produce heat

Traditional Moxibustion

Traditional Moxibustion therapy is the most practiced form of Moxibustion in contemporary Chinese clinics. It can be performed in two ways: directly, by placing Moxa onto the patient's body (this was once common practice), and indirectly, by burning it above or next to the affected area and releasing its medicinal effects through conduction heat transfer. Indirect Moxibustion can be used with various substances and herbs.

Drug Moxibustion

Drug Moxibustion employs irritant drugs (such as cantharis, semen Sinapis and pepper) to coat the skin around acupoints to make it flush or blistered. This process is often used to treat disease by stimulating local blood circulation.

Modern Moxibustion

Modern Moxibustion, like microwave and laser Moxibustion, has been developed to simulate traditional methods of applying heat (burning) or chemicals directly onto acupressure points. Practitioners use these new techniques to achieve therapeutic effects similar to those achieved through the at-home use of mugwort sticks (which can cause burns). Modern Moxibustion is considered safe and effective as long as it is performed by a trained professional. In addition to the traditional methods of burning incense over acupressure points, practitioners can also use laser-heated moxa sticks that emit infrared light (which heats the body).

Moxibustion Theories

Moxibustion employs materials like herbs and acupuncture points, which are burned to produce heat. The warmth generated by this method works differently than needles or drugs: Moxibustion's effects on the body have more to do with warming and nourishing. Warming and dredging are regarded as essential features of Moxibustion therapy.

Moxibustion can be used to expel cold from the body, boost circulation in meridians and collateral channels, clear away heat or dampness, and strengthen the immune system. Moxibustion's ability to arouse blood circulation and Qi flow groups it into warm nourishing, dredging, and melting.

Warm Nourishing

The effects of toning Qi (life energy), relieving depletion, and warming yang can be achieved by warm nourishing.

Warm Dredging

Warm dredging describes the effects of increased blood flow through the body and dissolving blockages. This promotes energy flow, drains excess fluids from tissues, relieves pain, and improves general health. Practitioners believe that Moxibustion's effectiveness stems from the warmth it generates. Moxibustion's purpose —is to expel cold, promote the circulation in meridians and collaterals, and clear away heat from an ailment (or dispel toxins).—is achieved through increased blood flow.

Warm Melting

The roles of warm-melting herbs are to remove phlegm, eliminate stagnation, dispel wind and dampness, draw out poisons and purify the blood. The basic theory of the Chinese is that the effects of Moxibustion are primarily based on the action of the meridian system.

The Meridian System

In traditional Chinese medicine, the meridian system is a concept that describes how energy flows through your body along specific pathways. The idea is that your body contains a network of energy pathways called meridians. Each meridian is associated with different organs or systems in your body and has specific functions. The meridian system is also responsible for regulating your health and well-being. By understanding how the meridians work, you can better understand how to use acupuncture as a healing tool. Moxibustion treatment acts on the body's nonspecific system of meridians, exerting its therapeutic effect through that mechanism.

Moxibustion is closely related to the meridian system, consisting of channels and collaterals. These pathways connect internal organs with external ones; they allow Qi (energy) and blood to flow throughout the body. Ling Shu determined twelve regular channels, the inner ones belonging to viscera and the outer ones connecting with limbs. According to TCM, a person is whole; therefore, illness manifests itself in one part of your body while having its root cause entirely elsewhere. The organs, limbs, and other body parts communicate with one another, and the rest of the body through an extensive network of pathways called meridians.

The twelve regular channels, known as cutaneous regions, are nourished by channel-qi. The skin is a reflection of the state of qi-blood flowing through meridians and organs and is responsive to treatment stimuli. Acupoints are the body surface locations where different organs and meridians concentrate their Qi. These points are target sites and response spots where treatment can be applied.

The skin regions and acupoints of the body are conduits through which Moxibustion's energy flows into the meridian system. Moxibustion can strengthen deficient conditions and reduce excessive ones, directly correcting the disease state of the body or activating its self-healing ability. For example, the different acupoints can treat many diseases through Moxibustion. Moreover, the same points have similar therapeutic effects regardless of whether they are treated by acupuncture or Moxibustion. These results prove that body meridians and acupoints are essential in treatment with this ancient Chinese medical technique.

Practicing Moxibustion

Acupuncturists use small needles made of various materials, like bamboo or stainless steel, combined with Moxa (herbs that create smoke when burned), depending on the direction desired to stimulate Qi flow. The Moxa is placed on the acupuncture point and held in place by a small, dampened piece of cotton. The acupuncturist will light the Moxa and let it burn for three to five minutes before discarding it. As the moxa burns, a practitioner will use glass cups or bowls to direct the smoke toward specific areas of the body.

The practice of Moxibustion is typically divided into three categories, each offering a different intensity level. These categories include:

Direct Scarring

Scarring Moxibustion uses a small cone of Moxa to burn an acupuncture point until the skin blisters. The affected area is allowed to heal on its own, typically over several months. The blisters can be removed at the end of this process, or they will fall off on their own.

Direct Non-Scarring

In direct non-scarring Moxibustion, the burning Moxa is removed before it has caused enough damage to the skin to leave a visible scar—unless too much time elapses between contact with and removal of the herb. It is also possible to use direct non-scarring Moxibustion to create a temporary burn, which eventually heals without leaving any scarring.

Indirect Moxibustion

Indirect Moxibustion, known as Oriental Baking or Chinese cupping, involves placing a cigar made of dried mugwort (Moxa) on the skin to heat it. The practitioner holds the cigar in place with one hand while inserting an acupuncture needle into another part of your body and gently moves them back and forth along its length. This motion causes blood vessels near the treated area to constrict temporarily so the Qi can be drawn closer to its source. Indirect Moxibustion is often used to treat chronic pain and inflammation. It also brings blood flow to the treated area, helping the body repair itself.

Stick on Moxa

This technique involves rolling a small amount of Moxa into thin pinches and lighting it on fire. Once fully ablaze, the moxa stick is placed directly onto one or more specific acupressure points along the body.

Moxa Wool

The practitioner salts the patient's navel kneads some wool into a cone shape, and places it on top of the salt. The size of the moxa wool varies depending on the treated condition; it can be small or large according to whether milder or stronger effects are needed.

Benefits of Moxibustion

Moxibustion is a form of acupuncture that uses heat to treat certain conditions by increasing blood circulation in the area. An acupuncturist targets specific areas of the body and triggers biochemical reactions that correspond to traditional meridian points. Moxibustion warms specific points of the body, producing heat that relieves muscle tension. The following are a few of the many benefits of Moxibustion.

- It improves blood flow and stimulates the body's natural healing processes.

- It removes cold and dampness from the body ("warming the meridians"), helping relieve pain in bones, muscles, tendons, and ligaments.

- Addresses female reproductive health issues, such as irregular menstrual cycles, infertility, and breech pregnancy

- Improves sexual health and fertility in men

- Resistance to cold and flu viruses is increased, making it easier for those repeatedly affected in the winter months

- Strengthens and boosts the immune system's ability to fight severe illnesses and keeps the body healthy

- Relaxes the muscles that line the digestive tract to normalize bowel movements

- Reduces tingling sensations in the fingers and toes

- Eliminates the risk of developing blood clots

- Reduces anxiety and alleviates specific symptoms of depression

- Mitigates the side effects of conventional cancer treatment

- Increases the flow of Qi throughout the body, resulting in an energized feeling that lasts all-day

- Promotes healthy joints and reduces pain associated with arthritis

- Improves the quality of sleep

- Reduces stress, tension, and anxiety

- Promotes a calmer state of mind

- It helps you fall asleep faster

Moxibustion and Herbs

Moxa is often used in conjunction with herbs and other substances. These can be mixed into the Moxa before use or burned separately on top of the Moxa. Materials used in Moxibustion are crucial, and their choice significantly affects its success. The following is a list of some common moxa and fire materials. It is by no means exhaustive, and the combination of herbs with other substances is also not limited to this list.

Ginger (Sheng Jiang)

Fresh ginger is cut into thin slices, and holes are made using a needle or a poking device. The slice is carefully placed on the desired acupuncture point. The Moxa cone is placed in the ginger and lit with a match. Once the Moxa becomes too hot, it is removed, and a fresh one is applied.

Garlic

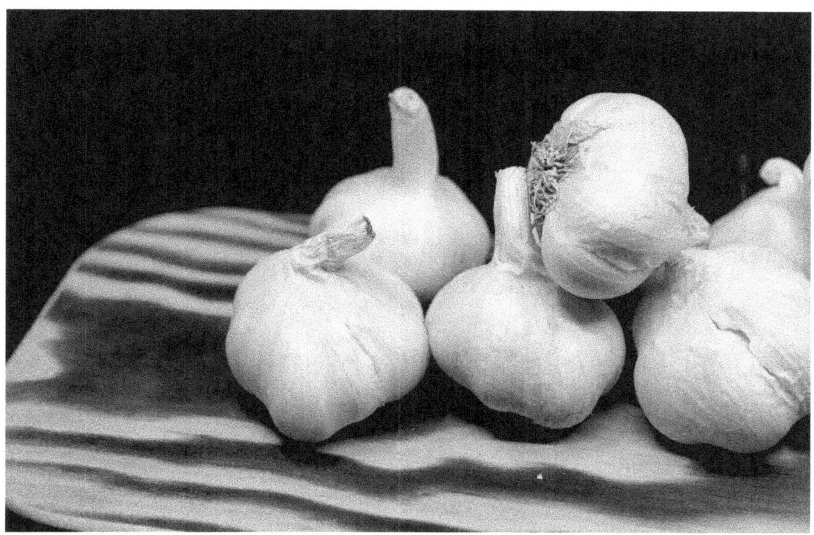

This method is similar to the one above and utilizes fresh garlic slices with numerous tiny holes. It treats specific acupuncture points or non-ulcerated carbuncles. It is customary to use three or eight Moxa cones during treatment, although more can be used if needed. The slice of garlic needs replacing every few minutes due to its potent properties when combined with the Moxibustion heat.

Blisters that develop in treated areas are common and should clear up after approximately one month (one acupuncture cycle).

Salt

A small amount of salt is poured into the navel and then topped with a slice of ginger. Moxa cones are placed on top to seal in the healing energy. This method is a restoring force to prevent the yang from collapsing.

Aconite (Fu Zi)

Fu Zi is a stiff, hard substance usually made into thin slices. It is placed on an Acupuncture point to relieve pain or illness. Moxa is placed in the center of Fu Zi and burned. Due to aconite's hot and spicy nature, this method can be used on any condition where yang is deficient. An alternative medium is grinding the Fu Zi root and mixing it with rice wine.

Pepper

This method involves grinding white pepper into a fine powder and combining it with flour before applying it to an acupuncture point. The moxa cone is placed on top of the powder, creating a slight depression in its center. This space can hold other herbs ground into smaller pieces, like cloves or cinnamon, before being inserted and ignited.

Moxa Rolls

Moxa rolls are made from dried and shredded herbs, ignited, and held in hand comfortably to provide heat to individual areas of the body. The stick is rubbed in a circular motion against the skin for 5 to 10 minutes or until the spot turns red. When applying intense stimulation, apply the stick to a particular part of the body and move it quickly from side to side.

Moxibustion and Safety

Moxibustion can be performed by a trained practitioner or by yourself at home. However, practicing it safely if you choose to do it yourself is essential. Here are some tips for practicing Moxibustion safely:

- Choose a clean location for your procedure, and ensure it is free from drafts or breezes that could blow the smoke away from your body and into your eyes or mouth

- Lay a towel under the treated area and reserve a small glass or ceramic dish for collecting any excess solution

- Hold one end of the Moxa stick above a flame source or gas stove

- Hold the lit end of the stick over an acupoint and keep it at an approximately one-centimeter distance from your skin so that no direct contact is made

- Move the stick back and forth in small, gentle motions. You should feel warmth without experiencing discomfort or sensation that is too hot to bear

- Brush ash from the end of the Moxa stick into its small dish so that it remains hot

- After Moxibustion has treated you, put the used Moxa stick in a jar with the lid tightly on to keep it from burning further

Most people can safely use Moxibustion, which is effective when done correctly. However, some safety issues must be considered before using Moxibustion as a treatment option:

- If you're pregnant or breastfeeding, talk to your doctor before using Moxibustion

- Don't use Moxa near your eyes or other sensitive areas of the body, like your stomach or groin area

- Don't use Moxa if you have an open wound or skin condition (such as psoriasis) or if taking blood thinners

- Stop using Moxa if you have abnormal bleeding, bruising, or swelling at the site where it was applied

- Don't perform Moxibustion on children or anyone with an open wound or skin infection. Perform it only on adults over 18 who have consented to receive treatment.

Chapter 6

Chinese Herbology

Chinese medicine is steeped in tradition and history, and herbs are crucial in its practices. They provide specific healing benefits and create balance within the body. This holistic approach is key to maintaining overall health and well-being. Traditional Chinese medicine utilizes thousands of different herbs, carefully selecting and combining them according to individual needs. These herbs can be ingested in various forms, including teas, pills, and tinctures.

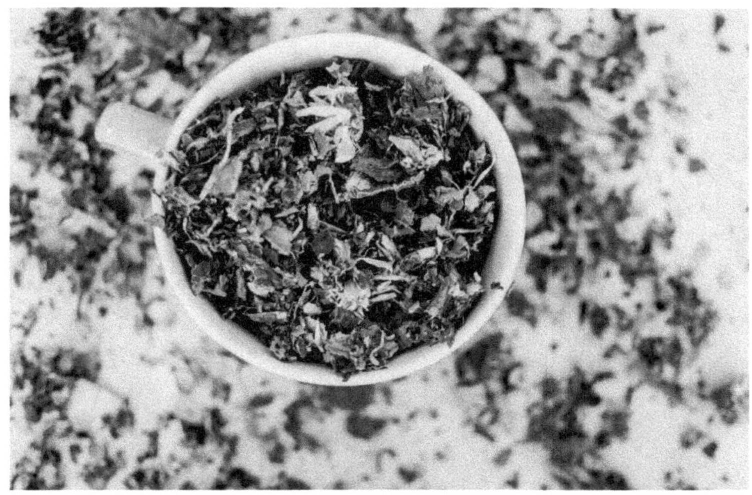

These herbs are often grown without chemicals and harvested at peak times to ensure quality and potency. While some Western medicine view herbs as an alternative or additional treatment, they provide significant relief from many conditions for many individuals. Herbs in Chinese medicine are deeply rooted in tradition and continue to show promising results in modern-day practices.

14 Important Herbs in Chinese Medicine

Chinese herbology uses many different herbs with unique properties and functions. It treats various conditions, ranging from the common cold to more serious diseases like cancer. While there are thousands of herbs used in Chinese medicine, here are 12 of the most important:

1. Angelica Root

Angelica root, known as dong quai or "female ginseng," is an herb used in Chinese medicine for centuries. It grows in the cold, damp mountain regions of China, Japan, and Korea. It is a celery family member with a long, thick root that is bright yellow on the inside. The plant has small, white flowers and large, feathery leaves.

Angelica root has been used for various purposes, including treating stomach issues, menstrual cramps, and fever. Angelica root is most commonly used in a decoction when the herb is simmered in water to make tea. Today, Angelica root is most commonly taken as a supplement.

The most common use of angelica root is to help treat menstrual cramps and other issues related to the female reproductive system. The purported benefits of angelica root are linked to its compounds, such as flavonoids, terpenes, and coumarins. These compounds have antioxidant, anti-inflammatory, and analgesic (pain-relieving) properties. Angelica root is sometimes combined with other herbal teas, such as ginger or chamomile, to enhance its effects. It can also be helpful for digestive issues like indigestion and constipation.

Angelica root is generally considered safe; it can cause side effects like skin irritation, upset stomach, and dizziness. Pregnant or breastfeeding women should not use Angelica root due to a lack of safety information.

2. Arnica

Arnica, known as Shan Jin Che, is a flowering herb belonging to the sunflower family. It grows in mountainous regions across Europe and North America. The plant is used in traditional Chinese medicine, dating back to the 1500s, to balance the yin and yang and tone the Qi (life force). Arnica has these effects because it helps to bring harmony between the different aspects of the body.

Arnica is most commonly used topically as an ointment or cream. In Chinese medicine, arnica treats various conditions, including bruises, muscle pain, and insect bites. It is applied to the skin for short periods, as prolonged exposure can irritate.

The leaves and flowers of the arnica plant are the parts most commonly used for medicinal purposes. Arnica contains helenalin, which is responsible for its anti-inflammatory effects. When applied to the skin, arnica gel or cream might decrease pain and swelling caused by injuries, surgery, and other conditions. It can be taken homeopathically in diluted forms and is sometimes used in hair tonics, anti-dandruff preparations, perfumes, and cosmetics. It treats mouth and throat inflammation and sores after dental surgery.

Arnica is typically soaked in alcohol to create a mixture, which is diluted and applied to skin disorders or injuries. It can also be consumed in very small amounts to provide pain relief. The plant is considered toxic if ingested and can cause vomiting, dizziness, and heart irregularities, and it should not be applied to broken skin. Additionally, contact with the plant can cause skin irritations. Arnica is also not recommended for pregnant women, as it is an abortifacient. It is best to consult a healthcare professional before using arnica, especially if you take other medications.

3. Celery

Celery (Apium graveolens or qin cai) is a member of the Apiaceae family, including carrots, parsley, and fennel. Celery is native to the Mediterranean region and has been used medicinally for centuries. The ancient Greeks and Romans utilized celery for its purported ability to ward off drunkenness and relieve joint pain. Celery is still used in traditional Chinese medicine for these purposes and also to treat high blood pressure and indigestion.

Celery can be eaten raw, cooked, juiced, or in supplement form. It is a good source of vitamins A, C, and K, folate, and potassium. Celery juice is especially beneficial, as it is a concentrated source of nutrients and antioxidants. Celery is often used to help treat conditions such as fevers, diarrhea, and hypertension.

Celery is generally considered safe to consume. However, some people may be allergic to celery or celery seed extract. If you experience any adverse effects after consuming celery, discontinue use and consult your doctor.

4. Cinnamon

Cinnamon is another popular herb in Chinese medicine that has been used for thousands of years. It comes from the bark of a cinnamon tree, and the chemical composition of the spice differs depending on the tree's species, and the part of the tree used. Two herbs in the Chinese materia medica are classified as cinnamon. The first is the Gui Zhi (cinnamon twig), and the second is Rou Gui (cinnamon tree bark).

Cinnamon twig in Chinese medicine is used to warm the meridians and relieve pain. It is often used for aches and pains associated with the common cold or flu and menstrual cramps. Cinnamon bark is more warming than a cinnamon twig and is used to treat colds and stomachaches.

Cinnamon has several health benefits, including the ability to:

- Boost cognitive function

- Reduce inflammation

- Fight infection

- Ease digestive issues

Cinnamon has antibacterial and antifungal properties and helps relieve nausea and vomiting. In addition, cinnamon can help regulate blood sugar levels, making it a good choice for people with diabetes.

Cinnamon is a safe spice, but it should be used in moderation. Too much cinnamon can lead to mouth sores, gastric upset, and diarrhea. Pregnant women or young children should not use cinnamon. If you have liver disease, consult with your doctor before using cinnamon.

5. Ginger

Ginger, known as shen Jiang, is a flowering plant that originated in China. Its botanical name is Zingiber officinale. The plant's underground stem (rhizome) is used for culinary or medicinal purposes. Ginger can be consumed in many ways, including fresh ginger, dried ginger, powder, capsules, and oil.

The Chinese use ginger to help with many different conditions, and it is often used in traditional Chinese medicine (TCM). In TCM, ginger is considered a "warming" herb to help circulation and treat stomach issues. It is also used as an anti-inflammatory agent. Ginger has many different benefits and can treat nausea, vomiting, and indigestion. It can also help relieve pain, reduce inflammation, and improve blood circulation.

A recent study showed that ginger is effective in treating osteoarthritis. The ginger extract significantly reduced pain and stiffness in knee osteoarthritis patients. Before taking ginger supplements, speak to your doctor about possible medication interactions.

6. Hawthorn Berry

Hawthorn berry, known as Shan Zha in Chinese, is a small, red fruit that grows on a thorny shrub. The hawthorn berry bush is found in many temperate regions worldwide and has been used for centuries in traditional Chinese medicine (TCM). It treats heart and blood vessel disorders such as congestive heart failure (CHF), chest pain, and irregular heartbeat. It is also used for digestive problems such as indigestion, diarrhea, and stomach pain.

The herb contains compounds that help expand blood vessels and improve blood flow, which improves heart function. It also helps stabilize blood pressure. In a 2006 study, Hawthorn Berry extract was found to be more effective than other medications in reducing diastolic blood pressure.

Another study showed that Hawthorn Berry could help improve inconsistent sleeping patterns and promote peaceful sleep due to the herb's calming effect on the nervous system.

Hawthorn berry is rich in antioxidants which help protect the body from damage caused by free radicals. This herb is also a good source of vitamins and minerals, including vitamin C, beta-carotene, calcium, and magnesium.

Hawthorn berries can take many forms, including capsules, tablets, tinctures, and tea. It is important to consult with a healthcare practitioner before taking any supplements, as Hawthorn berries can interfere with other medicines.

7. Ginkgo Biloba

Ginkgo Biloba (Yin Xing Ye) is a plant native to China. The leaves of the ginkgo Biloba tree are often used to make extract, which has various health benefits. After the leaves are dried, they are crushed into a powder. The powder can be taken orally or made into tea.

The main actions of ginkgo Biloba, according to traditional Chinese medicine, are: assisting the lung Qi, easing dyspnea and stopping coughing, activating blood circulation and eliminating blood stasis, and easing pain. It treats conditions such as dyspnea, coughing, hyperlipidemia, and angina.

Ginkgo Biloba extract increases blood flow to the brain, which helps improve cognitive function. The plant is also a powerful antioxidant; ginkgo Biloba's antioxidants help protect the brain from damage. Additionally, ginkgo Biloba has anti-inflammatory properties, contributing to its brain-protective effects.

Ginkgo Biloba should not be consumed together with seafood or fish. Additionally, ginkgo Biloba should be used with caution by people taking blood-thinning medications, as the plant could increase the risk of bleeding.

8. Licorice Root

Licorice (gan cao) is a plant found across Europe and Asia. Its root is commonly used for therapeutic and healing purposes. It has also been used to flavor food and as a sweetener for centuries because of its unique taste. Licorice root has many active compounds, the most important being glycyrrhizin and flavonoids.

Glycyrrhizin is an anti-inflammatory agent that also has antiviral properties. The effect is achieved by inhibiting the breakdown of cortisol. Cortisol is a stress hormone that helps the body deal with physical and emotional stress. When cortisol levels are too high, it can lead to anxiety, depression, and other health problems. Flavonoids help protect the body against damage from free radicals. Free radicals are molecules that can cause cell damage and lead to chronic diseases like cancer. Flavonoids also have anti-inflammatory and immune-boosting properties.

Licorice root is most commonly used to treat respiratory problems like bronchitis, cough, and sore throat. It is also used to treat stomach ulcers, heartburn, and indigestion. Licorice can be taken as capsules, tablets, tea, or tincture.

Licorice root is generally safe for most people when taken in small doses. However, it can cause side effects such as headaches, muscle pain, and water retention. It can also interact with certain medications, so it is important to talk to your doctor before taking licorice root. Pregnant women should not take licorice root because it can stimulate the uterus and lead to miscarriage. People with high blood pressure, kidney disease, or heart disease should also avoid taking licorice root.

9. Peppermint

Peppermint (bo he) is a plant originally from Europe. It is now found all across the world in temperate climates. Peppermint has been used medicinally for centuries to treat various conditions ranging from stomach pain to colds and flu.

The main active ingredient in peppermint is menthol. Menthol has been shown to have antiviral, antibacterial, and anti-inflammatory properties. It is also an effective decongestant and expectorant. Peppermint oil is commonly used in aromatherapy to relieve stress and tension headaches.

Peppermint is most commonly taken as a tea. To make peppermint tea, simply steep one teaspoon of dried peppermint leaves in boiling water for five minutes. You can also take peppermint oil capsules or drops (0.2-0.4 ml) daily.

Peppermint is generally safe and well-tolerated. Some people may experience heartburn or an upset stomach after taking peppermint. If this occurs, take peppermint with food or drink. Peppermint oil should not be taken internally by pregnant women or young children. Menthol can be toxic in large doses, so it is important to follow the recommended dosage.

10. Turmeric

Turmeric (Jiang Huang) is a dried rhizome of the Curcuma longa plant and is generally considered safe when used in small amounts as a spice. Turmeric's taste is bitter and pungent and targets the liver and spleen. In traditional Chinese medicine (TCM), the liver is often referred to as the body's "general" because it regulates the movements of Qi and body fluids, and turmeric helps restore the balance between them.

Turmeric can be used fresh, dried, or powdered. The fresh root is usually boiled and peeled before being eaten. The dried root can be ground into a powder and used as a spice. The powdered form is also used in supplements. Turmeric has many health benefits primarily due to curcumin's powerful anti-inflammatory and antioxidant effects.

Curcumin, the active ingredient in turmeric, is a powerful anti-inflammatory, effectively treating arthritis symptoms, such as pain and inflammation. Turmeric can help improve digestion and treat digestive disorders like irritable bowel syndrome (IBS). It prevents heart disease by reducing cholesterol levels and inflammation. Curcumin has been shown to inhibit the growth of cancerous cells and tumors. It also helps improve the effectiveness of chemotherapy drugs.

It reduces plasma levels of malondialdehyde and increases red blood cell catalase activity and plasma albumin levels in hemodialysis patients. Gargling with turmeric can delay and reduce the severity of mucositis in head and neck cancer patients undergoing radiation therapy.

When taken in small doses, turmeric is generally safe; however, there are a few contraindications to be aware of. Turmeric should be avoided during pregnancy and should not be used when there is Blood Deficiency with signs of Stagnumeric.

11. Milk Thistle

Milk thistle (Shui Fei Ji) is a flowering herb in the daisy family. It's native to Europe, North Africa, and Asia but is now found worldwide. The plant gets its name from the milky white sap that comes from its leaves when they're cut.

Milk thistle has been used for centuries as a natural remedy for various ailments. Today, it's most commonly taken as a supplement to help with liver and kidney problems. Some people also take milk thistles to help with kidney and digestive issues or to promote lactation.

Milk thistle is most commonly taken for liver problems. The active ingredient in milk thistle, silymarin, helps protect the liver from damage. Silymarin is a powerful antioxidant that helps detoxify the liver and repair it from damage caused by toxins.

In addition to its liver-protecting effects, milk thistle lowers blood pressure, regulates blood sugar levels, and helps with skin conditions like acne and psoriasis.

Milk thistle is available in many forms, including capsules, tablets, tinctures, and teas. It can also be found in foods like energy bars and shakes. The amount of milk thistle you should take depends on why you're taking it. So, you must follow the directions on the product.

Milk thistle is generally considered safe for most people. Some potential side effects include diarrhea, nausea, and bloating. Pregnant women should avoid milk thistle as it could stimulate menstruation. People with allergies to plants in the Asteraceae/Compositae family (daisies, marigolds, or chrysanthemums) should also avoid milk thistles.

12. Ginseng

Ginseng (Ren Shen) is a slow-growing plant with long, thick roots. It is native to East Asia but can now be found worldwide. Ginseng is most commonly used as a supplement but can also be found in some cosmetic products and energy drinks.

The two most common ginseng are Asian ginseng (Panax ginseng) and American ginseng (Panax quinquefolius). Depending on how it is processed, ginseng is sometimes referred to as red or white ginseng. Ginseng can be consumed in many different ways. It is commonly taken as a supplement in pill or capsule form. It can also be found in energy drinks, teas, and some cosmetic products.

Ginseng has a range of health benefits, including reducing stress and fatigue, boosting the immune system, and improving cognitive function. Natural treatments are sometimes used to treat sexual dysfunction and other health problems in men.

However, there is limited scientific evidence to support these claims, and ginseng can cause some side effects, such as insomnia, anxiety, and high blood pressure. Therefore, speaking to a healthcare provider before taking ginseng or any supplement is important.

13. Chamomile

Chamomile (Jin Zhen) is an herb commonly used in Chinese medicine. It is a member of the daisy family and has white and yellow flowers. Chamomile is native to Europe but can be found in other parts of the world. It has a long history of medicinal use and treats various conditions.

Chamomile is most commonly used to treat anxiety and insomnia but can treat other conditions. It has a calming effect on the body and helps treat stress.

Chamomile also treats digestive issues like upset stomach, diarrhea, and nausea. It can be found in many forms, including tea, capsules, and essential oils. It is generally considered safe for most people. However, it can interact with certain medications, so it is important to speak to a healthcare provider before taking it.

14. Schizandra

Schizandra (Wu Wei Zi) is a small, red berry native to China. Schizandra berries have a sweet and sour taste. The berries are dried and available in powder, capsule, or liquid form.

It is most commonly used as a supplement but is also used in some skincare products. It has various health benefits, including reducing stress, boosting energy levels, and improving skin complexion.

Schizandra is generally considered safe for most people, but it can interact with certain medications. Therefore, speaking to a healthcare provider before taking it is important.

There are many different schools of thought within Chinese herbology, but all practitioners believe in the importance of using natural substances to promote health and prevent disease. In Chinese herbology, the medical effects of herbs are often described in terms that reflect their physical appearance or traditional uses. These attributes can enhance the presentation and shelf life of infused waters. Understanding how these herbs work can create more interesting and efficacious products while increasing our marketability.

Chapter 7

Types of Remedies

Chinese herbal medicine is popular worldwide due to its effectiveness. People from all over Asia have sought these medicines as natural remedies for various ailments for centuries. The distinctiveness of Chinese medicine is evident in many applications, like depression or mood swings.

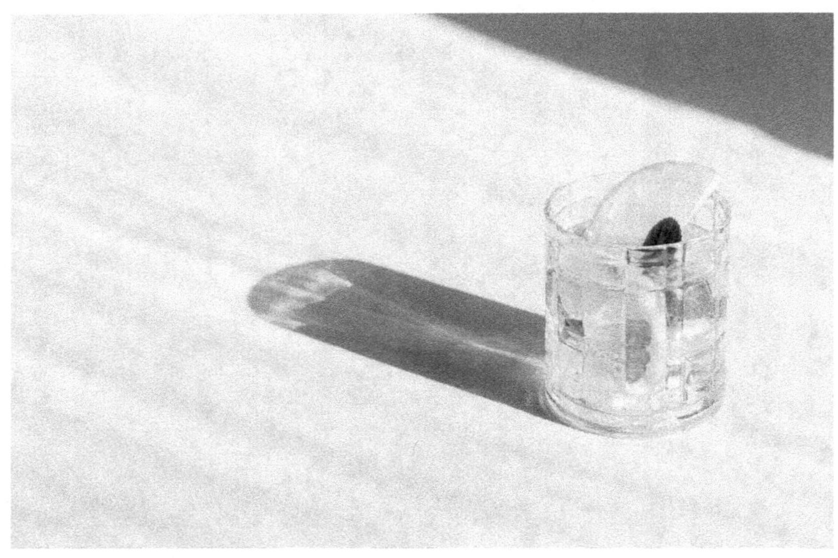

You might think some illnesses or discomforts have no cure, but Chinese medicine has solutions for most health issues, no matter how minor. This chapter teaches you about the various remedies in Chinese medicine, how to make them, and their potential applications. Each remedy is unique, and you can choose which one to use based on the materials available and the intended treatment.

Regardless of the remedy, consult a professional to ensure you select the right herb and preparation method to avoid abusing any herbs.

Decoctions

This involves the extraction of medicinal properties from hard roots, bark, dried berries, and seeds of plant materials by boiling them. Herbal medicines prepared in this manner have a stronger flavor. Medicines prepared by decoction are taken orally, but they can also be applied topically, generally, or in specific areas. This method of administration is common in Chinese herbal medicine.

They are quickly absorbed, so their action is the most potent compared to other traditional preparation methods. The formula is determined by the clinical need. Acute and serious conditions necessitate a specific decoction method.

When preparing your herbal medicine by decoction, keep in mind that a substantial amount of time will be required, especially for treating chronic diseases. Their flavor isn't always pleasant, but you can mask it with a sweetener like honey when necessary. Crush or grind the entire seed, bark, and root to extract the medicinal properties fully.

To make a decoction, place all the herbs in a pot and add twice as much water as the herbs. Heat for 30 minutes and ensure the pot is tightly closed to avoid evaporation of essential constituents. After boiling, remove from heat and strain through a filter. The decoction is ready to use and can be taken on its own or mixed with other medicines. However, you should consult with a professional before you begin.

There is also a dried decoction form known as syrup, which is produced by evaporating the liquid after it has been strained using a vacuum and heat. The syrup is dried further using a spray drier and a powder carrier until it forms a powder. You can make do with liquid decoction because dried decoction requires a lot of technicalities.

Root decoction can treat breathing difficulties, muscle spasms, and bladder or kidney inflammation. Understanding that the herbs gathered are determined by the illness being treated is critical. You must obtain your prescription from a qualified and practicing Chinese medical professional.

Each root, bark, or seed has a unique medicinal property, and the proper combination of herbs is required to achieve the desired effect. For centuries, people have used Suanzaoren decoction to treat insomnia. The Shaoyao-Gancao decoction has been used for many years in Asia to treat dysmenorrhea and abdominal pain.

Infusion

Infusion should be your preferred preparation method if you want to get all of the flavor and oil your favorite herbs offer. Most people prefer this method because of its medicinal value or the distinct taste it gives the finished product. In this method, the selected herbs are steeped in cold or hot water for the sufficient time it takes for the water to absorb the flavor and oil from the herbs.

Herbal teas are also considered infusions because they are soaked in water to extract the medicinal component. The primary distinction between herbal tea and a proper herbal infusion is that tea infusion uses herbal leaves, whereas proper infusion uses flowers, leaves, shoots, and roots. The steeping time for tea is short, limiting the number of nutrients that can be obtained. A proper herbal infusion can take up to 24 hours to produce the desired results, especially if cold water is used. Infusions are regarded as a safe and natural way to consume herbs.

As previously stated, some people choose infusion for its great flavor and taste rather than its medicinal value. Herbal infusions are simple to prepare, and the purpose of the treatment determines which herbs should be combined and how long the infusion process should last.

Unique herbs steeped at different times have different nutritional benefits. Certain herbs taste better when steeped longer. Hot herbal infusion aids in the extraction of volatile aromatic oil, enzymes, and vitamins from aromatic roots, leaves, and flowers. Cold herbal infusion extracts essential oil and medicinal constituents from mucilaginous herbs; however, infusing herbs in cold water takes more time to extract the medicinal components. Infusions do not last long, especially when cold water is used; they could last a couple of days but should immediately be discarded if you notice a change in flavor, color, or taste.

To make an infusion, steep dried or powdered herbs in cold or boiling water overnight or until drinkable. Use a glass jar with a tight lid to avoid nutrient loss due to evaporation. Ensure to cover the herbs completely with boiling water. The duration of the infusion is determined by the herb and the amount of extract expected. Using a strainer, remove the liquid while ensuring no herb remains in the infusion. Use cheesecloth to make the straining process easier.

Aloe vera infusions can help with irritable bowel syndrome, constipation, and ulcerative colitis. Mint infusions relieve gas, soothe an upset stomach, and prevent vomiting and nausea. Gargling thyme infusion can treat mouth sores and bad breath. Chamomile infusions help calm anxiety and insomnia.

Identifying the medical issue to address is the bottom line in determining which infusion to make. You must select the appropriate herb for the infusion based on the circumstances. It is best to seek professional assistance before making an herbal infusion to avoid doing it incorrectly and jeopardizing your health.

Soaks

Soaking in Chinese medicine has been used to exfoliate the skin and eliminate external invaders for years. The herbal SPA involves immersing yourself in hot herbal solutions tailored to specific health concerns.

The herbs used for soaking should be prescribed by an herbalist, and excessive use should be avoided, especially if not directed by your physician. Essential oils have been used for centuries for relaxation and skin care; to maximize their beneficial effects, add a few drops to a hot bath before soaking.

Herbal soaks can be made with traditional herbs such as lavender, ylang-ylang, jasmine, oat-top ginger, cleavers, orange fir, grapefruit, geranium, rosemary, peppermint, calendula, chamomile, and rose. Other interesting ingredients for spa treatments include bath oil, pink salt, sea salt, and Epsom salt. After soaking, spray your skin with rose, blood orange, lime, or peppermint.

To make home soaks, mix baking soda and salt and add half to a tub of hot water. Add a few drops of essential oil and allow the soda and salt to dissolve before getting in. Some herbs are used to soak the feet to relax muscles and relieve stress. Choose essential oils or herbs that suit your mood - for example, if you feel stressed, add lavender. Do you want a calming fragrance? Add geranium or sweet orange to the mix. Are you looking for something to relax your muscles? Rosemary is ideal.

Herbal SPA helps with detoxification by increasing sweat secretion and toxin metabolism. Soaking improves blood circulation, meridian circulation, and lymph circulation. It also aids in restoring endocrine balance, preventing diseases, and increasing immunity, which contributes to a longer lifespan.

Soaking is beneficial for postpartum repair, treating skin diseases, preventing cerebrovascular and cardiovascular diseases, and moisturizing the skin. It also helps digestion and gastrointestinal movement. Additionally, it helps you relax and sleep better.

Compresses

Herbal compresses are traditional Chinese medicines used to treat a variety of ailments. It entails massaging the herbal compress into the affected areas. This therapy can be applied to soft tissues like fascia and muscles to help relieve stress, improve blood circulation, promote overall health, improve sleep, and stimulate the lymphatic system for proper waste removal.

It also treats shoulder, neck, and lower-back pain. A masseur will use this herbal compress to massage your entire body or specific areas, like traditional Thai massage. The compress comprises various herbs wrapped in muslin cloth. The muslin cloth is tightly rolled up and steamed until it is piping hot. The therapist or masseur will directly pound or press the compress against your skin. Depending on your needs, the compress is concentrated on your shoulders, neck, or entire body.

To make this compress, start with a goal and use that to determine which herbs to combine and how much to use. Gather the herbs in the center of a porous cloth because the steam and herbal droplet must pass through the cloth and penetrate the skin. Fold the edges of the cloth together to form a tight round ball. Tie a thread around the top of the compress to make a handle. Ensure to tie the compress firmly so it doesn't come undone during use. Steam the herbal compress for at least 30 minutes and check the temperature with your inner forearm. It should not be too hot to touch. Using the compressed ball, massage and pound the area of interest.

This method can relieve aches, tension, and muscle pain. It is also an excellent lymphatic system stimulant, increasing blood circulation and flow. Herbs differ in their properties and health benefits. For example, cumin helps treat diarrhea and fight parasites and bacteria, and camphor trees help relieve pain, improve breathing, and treat certain skin conditions.

Tamarind detoxifies the body and is beneficial for treating heart disease, diabetes, and cancer. Turmeric is used for detoxification and also has anti-inflammatory properties. There are far too many benefits to list, so incorporate massage compresses into your SPA treatment.

Capsules

Capsules are medications with an outer shell. The outer shell is easily broken down in your digestive tract, allowing the medication to be absorbed into your bloodstream. Using capsules as traditional medicines may seem implausible, but the active medicinal component of a plant can be isolated and packaged inside a capsule for more efficient administration.

Hard-shelled capsules are ideal for extended-release and dual-action formulas. To create an enclosed casing, insert one half of the capsule into the other. The inner shell contains dry pellets or powdered medication, and the outer shell contains liquid medication. Soft-gel capsules contain medication suspended in gelatin.

Capsulized herbal remedies provide rapid relief from illnesses. If you find the taste of certain herbal medicines unpleasant, taking them as capsules will be beneficial. Making capsules require professional and technical skills you might lack, so seeking help from experts in this field is important.

Certain herbs can be capsulated. These include valerian root powder, turmeric, triphala, spirulina, saw palmetto, hydrangea, horsetail, damiana, cranberry, chlorella, cayenne, black walnut, and ashwagandha. To make a capsule from any of the herbs mentioned above, you must powder them, as only powdered herbs should be encapsulated.

Each plant has its distinct medicinal property - for example, damiana leaf powder's ability to stimulate sexual desire was traditionally used in various cultures. Additionally, damiana can improve mood, stimulate digestion, and promote relaxation.

Turmeric capsules are derived from turmeric roots and help promote healthy joint movement. These herbs can be purchased in the form of leaves, roots, seeds, or bark; however, before encapsulation, the herbs must be ground into a fine powder, regardless of which form it comes in.

When making your first homemade herbal capsule, you'll need powdered herbs, empty shells made from a plant-based source, a capsule machine to aid mass production, a shallow glass dish to collect capsules as you produce them, and a glass jar for storage. The herb you encapsulate must be based on your medical needs.

Liniments

Liniments are herbal remedies that aid in relieving soft tissue and muscle pain. This remedy is produced with alcohol, allowing it to absorb through the skin easily. Liniments are made by combining herbs of significant medicinal importance.

Menthol is a member of the mint family and is used to make soothing and cooling liniments. Liniments made from Hypericum perforatum (St. John's Wort) treat nerve pain, injured soft tissues, and overworked muscles.

Liniments are alcohol-based remedies made by soaking herbs in alcohol for an extended period; using alcohol facilitates skin penetration. If the herbs used are oil-rich, the alcohol will aid in extracting those oils. Liniments are very useful for athletes, martial artists, and physically active people for an extended period.

Capsicum frutescens relieves pain by blocking pain transmission messages to your brain. It makes liniments for achy and sore muscles, joint pains, and arthritis. Arnica increases blood flow and circulation to injured areas; however, it should not be used on open wounds.

Chamomile liniment is excellent for relieving pain, reducing inflammation, and healing wounds. This remedy can be prepared to treat numerous joint and muscle pains. It also heals damaged bones, tissues, and inflamed cells. There are specific herbs for various ailments, and you can combine a couple of herbs for the best results.

After determining the ailment to be treated and the herbs required, coarsely grind the dried herbs using a pestle and mortar and place them in an airtight pint jar. Pour alcohol into the jar through the opening at the top. Allow this mixture to sit for at least four weeks. Shake the jar daily during the steeping period, strain the herb, add essential oil, transfer the mixture into a suitable container, and use.

Apply the liniment to the wounded area, but make sure it is not an open wound. Massage it into your skin, and allow it to penetrate and release its healing effect.

Herbal Teas

Herbal medicines have been used to save lives for centuries. People from across the world rely on Chinese herbal medicine to meet their various healthcare needs. Despite advances in technology and conventional medicine, people still rely heavily on herbal remedies.

Some individuals use herbal medicines because they are inexpensive and widely available, while others use them because of their personal health ideology. Many people drink herbal tea daily for various health reasons, and we will look at some herbs that are great for teas in this section.

Ginseng

This herb in traditional Chinese medicine boosts immunity, increases energy, improves brain function, and reduces inflammation. To make this tea, steep the herb's root in hot water. Ginseng comes in two varieties: American ginseng and Asian ginseng, which promote relaxation and stimulation.

Ginseng tea is made by steeping a ginseng tea bag in hot water, allowing it to cool to a drinkable temperature, straining it, and then drinking. The tea bag contains raw ground ginseng bagged for convenience.

Ginkgo Biloba

Ginkgo Biloba has been used in Chinese herbal medicines for centuries, and its popularity is growing. This herbal tea is made from the leaves and seeds of the plant. Blend the dried leaves and infuse the nutrients in a cup of hot water for a few minutes before drinking. Since the seed is mildly toxic, use it in small quantities.

This herbal tea treats sexual dysfunction, mental issues, dementia, and heart diseases. Increased bleeding risk, skin reaction, digestive issues, heart palpitations, and headaches are among the side effects.

Regardless of this tea's numerous benefits, drink it in moderation and as directed by your doctor or herbalist.

Peppermint

This mint tea is widely consumed around the world for many health reasons. Peppermint tea has antiviral and antibacterial properties and anticancer, antioxidant, and digestive tract support. Enjoy a cup of peppermint tea the next time you have indigestion, nausea, or cramping.

Raspberry Leaves

Raspberry tea is made by steeping raspberry leaves in hot water. This traditional Chinese herbal tea relieves pregnancy symptoms like cramping and diarrhea. It also contains powerful antioxidants such as flavonoids, tannin, and vitamin E. Red raspberry leaves can also be used to make tea to treat throat and mouth inflammation, diarrhea, and mild cramps.

Elderberry

This is a Sambucus nigra plant with numerous health benefits. You can make an herbal tea with elderberry, ginger, and honey. It aids in treating common colds and flu. Avoid eating raw or unripe elderberry fruits because they are toxic and can cause vomiting, diarrhea, or nausea.

St. John's Wort

The herb St. John's Wort is derived from the flowering plant Hypericum perforatum. It has small yellow flowers commonly used to make tea and other drinks. This herbal tea is useful for treating various conditions, including depression, insomnia, lung and kidney diseases, and injuries.

Dry mouth, photosensitivity, confusion, dizziness, and allergic reactions are some of its side effects. Overdosing on this tea is unhealthy, so drink moderately. If you're on medication, consult your doctor before taking this tea.

Ginger

This herbal tea has treated high blood pressure, nausea, migraines, and colds for centuries. Ginger tea relieves nausea in pregnant women and cancer patients. It has few side effects, but overdosing can cause diarrhea and heartburn.

Valerian

Once it has been dried, this herb's root can make tea by steeping it in hot water for a few minutes. Valerian has recently been used to treat anxiety and insomnia. It induces sleep, so avoid drinking this tea if you take sedatives to avoid compounding effects.

In Chinese medicine, dozens of herbs are used as herbal tea. Your goals determine the tea. Herbal teas are simple to prepare and serve as a morning routine to start your day. If you drink herbal tea, don't overdo it. Moderation in medications is essential, particularly herbal medicines.

Chinese medicines have many effective applications. Traditional Chinese medicine is self-sufficient due to its versatility. It addresses all aspects of health care while remaining accessible and affordable. The nature of the illness will determine the remedy.

Each remedy's constituents are extracted differently; some herbs work well in combination with other related herbs, while others work well on their own. You cannot administer some treatments yourself, like the compress massage; however, you can replace this with soaking. The most important thing is to find efficient herbs for your required treatment. The remedies mentioned in this chapter will help you find the best one.

Chapter 8

Remedies for Anxiety

Everyone experiences anxiety at some point in their lives. However, some individuals experience extreme cases of anxiety that disrupts their daily life. Some medications are known to relax anxiety symptoms, but many avoid them due to certain side effects. That's where herbal remedies come in handy.

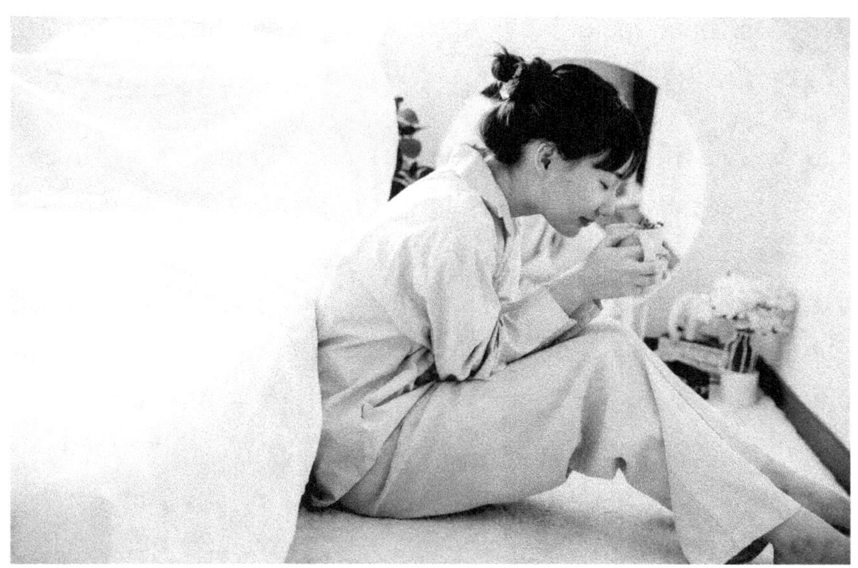

Traditionally, Chinese medicine practitioners also believe that good health is the result of a balance between yin and yang. These are two opposite but interconnected forces that are present in all things. When these forces are in balance, a person is in good health. However, when yin and yang become imbalanced, it can lead to illness. According to traditional Chinese medicine (TCM), anxiety is caused by an imbalance between yin and yang.

Shan You Si is a traditional Chinese medicine term that refers to stress and anxiety disorders. According to TCM, these disorders are caused by imbalances in the Zang organs, which include the heart, lungs, spleen, and kidneys. Treatment for Shan You Si typically involves acupuncture, herbal remedies, and lifestyle changes. For example, patients may be advised to eat a healthy diet, exercise regularly, and get enough sleep. TCM practitioners believe that Shan You Si can be effectively treated by restoring balance to the Zang organs.

If you're one of those people, you may be looking for ways to cope with your anxiety. Traditional Chinese Medicine (TCM) herbs have been used for centuries to treat a variety of conditions, including anxiety. Many different herbs can be used to treat anxiety, each with its own unique benefits. Herbs can help to calm the mind and body, relieve stress, and promote relaxation. In addition, herbs can be used to regulate the flow of qi, or life energy, within the body. When qi is unbalanced, it can lead to feelings of anxiety and unease. By restoring balance to the body's qi, herbs can help to reduce anxiety and promote a sense of well-being. While TCM herbs can be effective in treating anxiety, it's important to choose and mix the right herb to contain the effects of anxiety. Here are some of the main herbs used in traditional Chinese medicine which can help you manage your anxiety and live a more peaceful life.

1. Polygonum Root- Hu Zhang

Hu Zhang (Polygonum cuspidatum) is a traditional Chinese medicinal herb used for centuries to treat various ailments, including anxiety. The active ingredients in polygonum root, like nerve growth factor and piperine, effectively reduce anxiety and promote relaxation. In addition, polygonum root is a rich source of antioxidants and anti-inflammatory compounds, which help protect the body from the damaging effects of stress. Much research confirms the efficacy of polygonum root for treating anxiety, and its long history in traditional Chinese medicine suggests it is a helpful natural treatment for this condition.

Polygonum root has a calming effect on the body and is often prescribed for patients experiencing stress or having difficulty sleeping. Polygonum root is sometimes combined with other herbs, such as ginger or ginseng, to enhance its effects further. While no scientific evidence supports using polygonum root for anxiety, many people find it helps relieve their symptoms.

In recent years, scientific research has confirmed many of the therapeutic effects of Hu Zhang, and it is now considered one of the most important hepatoprotective and cholagogic drugs in traditional Chinese medicine (TCM). Hu Zhang contains a number of active constituents that contribute to its therapeutic effects, including resveratrol, quercetin, and emodin. These compounds have been shown to protect the liver from damage by toxins, improve bile flow, and lower cholesterol levels. In addition, Hu Zhang has been effective in treating hypertension, hyperlipidemia, and cardiovascular and neurodegenerative diseases.

2. Jujube Fruits - Hong Zhao

Jujube fruits, botanically classified as Ziziphus jujuba, are small, round drupes that grow on deciduous trees belonging to the Rhamnaceae family. Native to China, these popular fruits have been cultivated for over 4,000 years. They have spread to many parts of Asia and the Mediterranean. Jujubes are often used in traditional Chinese medicine (TCM) and are known as hong zao in Mandarin.

These unique fruits are available in two main varieties: Indian jujube and Chinese red date. Indian jujubes are typically smaller and softer than Chinese red dates, which are larger and have a harder texture. Both varieties can be eaten fresh or dried and used in a variety of culinary applications, such as jams, jellies, candies, pies, pastries, soups, stews, and tea.

Jujube fruits are an excellent source of vitamins C and B2 and contain high dietary fiber levels. In TCM, jujube fruits have calming properties and treat anxiety, insomnia, and indigestion. They also boost energy levels and improve circulation. Whether eaten fresh or used in traditional medicine, jujube fruits offer a wide range of benefits.

According to TCM, anxiety is caused by an imbalance of yin and yang energies in the body. Jujube fruits help restore this balance, as they are relatively neutral in nature. In addition to their calming effects, jujube fruits boost the immune system and improve digestion. For these reasons, they are often taken as a tonic or tea before bedtime. There are several different ways jujube fruits can treat anxiety, depending on the severity of the condition. Jujube fruits contain compounds that help regulate the body's stress response. In particular, jujube fruits effectively reduce cortisol levels, a hormone released in response to stress. Additionally, jujube fruits contain antioxidants to protect the body from the damaging effects of stress.

Therefore, the scientific evidence supports using jujube fruits in TCM for treating anxiety. For mild anxiety, jujube tea can be drunk three times daily. For more moderate cases of anxiety, jujube pills or powder can be taken three times daily. For severe cases of anxiety, jujube extract can be taken three times daily. Jujube fruits are safe and effective for treating anxiety and can be found at most health food stores.

3. Rehmanniae

Rehmanniae is a Chinese herbal medicine. The Chinese name for Rehmanniae is Sheng Di Huang, meaning "raw land yellow." Rehmanniae is classed as an herb that clears heat and cools the blood. In traditional Chinese medicine (TCM), Rehmanniae can help treat a number of conditions, including fever, headaches, fatigue, and bruising. Rehmanniae is typically used in a decoction, meaning they are boiled in water to extract the active ingredients. The herb is sometimes combined with other ingredients, like licorice root or white peony root, to enhance its effects. People taking Rehmanniae must be aware that it can cause gastrointestinal upset, so it is important to start with small doses and increase gradually.

One of the most commonly used herbs is Rehmanniae, which effectively treats anxiety. There are several explanations for why this herb is helpful in treating anxiety. First, Rehmanniae has a calming effect on the mind and body. It could be due to its rosmarinic acid content, which has had anti-anxiety effects in animal studies. Additionally, Rehmanniae is a rich source of antioxidants and has anti-inflammatory properties. These properties help protect against the negative effects of stress on the body, including anxiety. Finally, Rehmanniae stimulates the production of GABA, a neurotransmitter vital in regulating anxiety. These properties, taken together, suggest that Rehmanniae is an effective treatment for anxiety.

It is often combined with other herbs, like Poria cocos and Codonopsis pilosula, to create a formula tailored to the individual's specific needs. Rehmanniae can be taken in many different forms, including decoctions, powders, tinctures, and capsules. The most important thing is to determine what works well for you and to take it regularly. While Rehmanniae is very effective in treating anxiety, remember that it is only one part of a comprehensive treatment plan. Other lifestyle changes, like regular exercise and eating a healthy diet, are also important for managing anxiety.

4. Polyrachis Ant- Ma Yi

Polyrachis Ant, known as "big-head ant," has been used in traditional Chinese medicine (TCM) for centuries. Also known as "chonglou," these ants are prized for their abilities to tonify the blood and promote circulation. They are often used to treat conditions like anemia and women's health issues. Polyrachis ants are also used to boost energy levels and immunity. In addition, they have anti-aging properties. Polyrachis ants are available in various forms, including capsules, powders, and liquids. Generally, they are considered safe, but it is always best to consult a qualified TCM practitioner before taking any supplements.

Polyrachis Ant is a traditional Chinese medicine to treat anxiety for centuries. The active ingredient in Polyrachis Ant is an alkaloid called pyrrolidine, which has sedative and hypnotic effects. In a recent study, pyrrolidine was found to be as effective as diazepam (Valium) in reducing anxiety in rats. Additionally, Polyrachis Ant does not appear to interact with other medications or cause any significant side effects. The ant is rich in nutrients and has a high protein content, making it an ideal herbal remedy for those with anxiety. Polyrachis Ant calms the nerves and improves blood circulation. Therefore, it could be an effective option for those seeking an alternative to traditional anxiety medications. The ant is often consumed in tea, capsule, tinctures, and extracts. For those with anxiety, Polyrachis Ant is an effective and safe herbal remedy that can help improve overall health and well-being.

5. Duanwood Reishi

Duanwood Reishi, known as "The Great Protector," is a medicinally valuable mushroom used in traditional Chinese medicine for centuries. Also known as Lingzhi or Ganoderma lucidum, this mushroom grows on the trunks of hardwood trees, typically in Northeast China. The mushroom's fruiting body is large and flat, with a bright red or orange color. Duanwood Reishi has a long history in TCM, where it is prized for its ability to tonify the liver and kidneys, calm the mind, and boost immune function. Modern scientific research has shown that Duanwood Reishi contains various compounds with medicinal properties, including polysaccharides, triterpenes, and ganoderic acids. As a result, this mushroom is now used as a natural remedy for a wide range of conditions, including insomnia, anxiety, and chronic fatigue.

In TCM, anxiety is often caused by an imbalance of yin and yang energy in the body. The Duanwood Reishi mushroom helps restore this balance, calm the mind, and ease stress. Duanwood mushrooms contain compounds that help regulate the serotonin levels in the brain. Serotonin is a neurotransmitter that stimulates mood and anxiety. By regulating serotonin levels, Duanwood Reishi helps reduce symptoms of anxiety. In addition, the mushroom contains compounds that help reduce inflammation. Chronic inflammation has been linked to anxiety and other mental health conditions. Duanwood Reishi improves overall mental health by reducing inflammation.

There are several ways to consume Duanwood Reishi for anxiety relief. One popular method is tea by boiling the mushrooms in water. It can be taken daily or as needed. Another option is Duanwood Reishi capsules, readily available at many health food stores. Some people also add these mushrooms to soups or other dishes. Regardless of how it is consumed, the Duanwood Reishi mushroom is an effective natural remedy for anxiety.

6. Ginseng

Ginseng is a plant used for its medicinal properties for centuries. The Chinese name for ginseng is Ren Shen, meaning "root of man" because it looks like a human body. Ginseng is used in traditional Chinese medicine (TCM) to help with many different ailments. Some include fatigue, anxiety, stress, improving cognitive function and memory, and boosting the immune system.

As a remedy for anxiety, ginseng effectively regulates the immune response and hormonal changes due to stress, maintaining homeostasis and curing anxiety. Ginseng has been shown to reduce cortisol levels, the stress hormone. Cortisol is responsible for the fight-or-flight response, and when levels are chronically high, it can lead to anxiety and other health problems. Ginseng also enhances the adrenal gland functions, which help regulate stress hormones. In addition, ginseng stimulates the production of natural killer cells, which is important for immunity and attacking cancer cells. The active ingredients in ginseng, called ginsenosides, are responsible for its many health benefits. Ginseng is safe for most people to take, but it can cause some side effects like insomnia and headaches. Ginseng is an effective natural remedy for anxiety and stress when taken as directed.

Ginseng can be consumed in several ways to treat anxiety, and the most common method is tea. To make a ginseng tea, boil water to steep slices of fresh ginseng root or dried ginseng powder. Once the ginseng has steeped in hot water for 3-5 minutes, add honey or sugar for sweetness. Some people also add other herbs to the tea, such as chamomile or lemon balm, both known for their calming effects. Another way to consume ginseng is as a supplement in pill form. Ginseng supplements are widely available in health food stores and online and can be taken daily to help reduce anxiety. Choosing a high-quality supplement made with pure ginseng extract is imperative for best results. Talking to a healthcare professional before taking ginseng is important, as it can interact with medications. Overall, ginseng is a safe and effective herb with many benefits.

7. Dang Gui

Danggui, or Chinese Angelica, is a root used in traditional Chinese medicine (TCM). It is sweet and pungent and nourishes blood, and moistens dryness. The botanical name for Danggui is Angelica sinensis, sometimes called Tang Kuei, Dong Quai, or Chinese Angelica. In TCM, the blood is considered the "mother" of Qi or vital energy, which nourishes the organs, tissues, and body cells, so it is not surprising that herbs that nourish blood are highly prized in this medicine system. Common uses of danggui include pain relief from menstrual cramps, and menopause symptoms such as hot flashes, night sweats, anxiety, and fatigue. It also treats digestive issues like diarrhea, constipation, indigestion, anemia, and irregular menstruation. Danggui's purported ability to cleanse the blood has led to its use in skin care products for conditions like acne, eczema, and psoriasis.

Dang Gui is a prolific flowering plant in the family Apiaceae and is native to Asia. The plant's roots are commonly used in traditional Chinese medicine (TCM) as a treatment for anxiety. Dang Gui has been shown to reduce anxiety in animal studies effectively. It increases gamma-aminobutyric acid levels (GABA) in the brain. GABA is a neurotransmitter that helps regulate nerve activity. Low levels of GABA are associated with anxiety and stress. Dang Gui also affects other neurotransmitters, including serotonin and dopamine, regulating mood. In addition to its effects on neurotransmitters, Dang Gui also has anti-inflammatory and antioxidant properties. These properties contribute to its ability to reduce anxiety.

Dang Gui can be consumed to treat anxiety in many ways, depending on the specific ingredients and proportions. A popular recipe combines Dang Gui with ginger, jujube fruit, and rice wine. Another variation adds licorice root and thinly sliced fresh ginger to boiled Dang Gui root - this mixture is taken orally two or three times a day. Generally, Dang Gui effectively relieves anxiety by promoting circulation and balancing the nervous system. When selecting a recipe or preparation method, consulting a qualified TCM practitioner to ensure the correct ingredients and proportions is crucial.

8. Xiao Yao Powder

Xiao Yao Powder is a traditional Chinese medication that has been in use for centuries. The powdered form of the herb is made from the plant's dried leaves, which is native to China. The leaves are ground into a fine powder and then ingested. Xiao Yao Powder is said to help with a variety of health conditions, including anxiety, depression, insomnia, and stress. It is also believed to boost energy levels, improve circulation, and promote healthy skin. While no scientific evidence supports these claims, many people find that taking Xiao Yao Powder helps them feel better overall. If you are interested in trying this remedy, be sure to purchase it from a reputable source.

TCM practitioners have long used Xiao Yao Powder to treat anxiety. The ingredients in the powder are said to nourish the liver and spleen, two organs that play an important role in regulating emotions. The liver is responsible for storing blood and maintaining the free flow of qi, while the spleen is responsible for Transformation and Transportation of Qi and Blood. When both organs function properly, they help keep the mind calm and balanced. However, when they are out of balance, it can lead to feelings of anxiety and restlessness. Xiao Yao Powder is thought to help restore balance by providing the liver and spleen with the nutrients they need to function properly. In addition to its calming effects, Xiao Yao Powder is also said to boost energy levels and improve digestion. As a result, it is often used as part of a comprehensive treatment plan for anxiety.

The powdered form of the herb is typically taken with water, but it can also be combined with other liquids or taken dry. Xiao Yao Powder can also be added to food or taken in capsule form. When taken as directed, Xiao Yao Powder is generally safe and well-tolerated. Some people may experience mild side effects such as upset stomach, headaches, or dizziness. If you experience any severe side effects, consult your healthcare provider.

9. Licorice Root

For those struggling with anxiety, the prospect of finding an effective treatment can feel daunting. However, several options are available, including traditional Chinese medicine (TCM). One popular herb used in TCM is licorice root. Licorice root is a type of herb that is commonly used in Traditional Chinese Medicine (TCM). The scientific name for licorice root is Glycyrrhiza glabra. It is also known by its Chinese name, Gan Cao. Licorice root is often used as a flavoring agent in food and beverages, but it also has a number of medicinal uses. In TCM, licorice root is thought to be sweet and neutral in nature. It is believed to have properties that can help to harmonize other herbs and ingredients in a formula. As a result, it is often used as a base ingredient in many different types of herbal formulas. Licorice root is thought to have several health benefits, including treating stomach ulcers, bronchitis, and genital herpes. It can also be used as a laxative and an expectorant. In addition, some people believe that licorice root can help to boost immunity and increase energy levels. While more research is needed to confirm these purported benefits, there is no doubt that licorice root has been used medicinally for centuries.

In traditional Chinese medicine, licorice root is commonly used to treat various conditions, including anxiety. While the exact mechanism is not fully understood, the herb is thought to work by regulating levels of the hormone cortisol in the body. Cortisol is often referred to as the "stress hormone" because it is released in response to stressful situations. This release can cause a number of symptoms, including anxiety and irritability. By regulating cortisol levels, licorice root may help to reduce these symptoms. In addition, the herb is thought to possess antioxidant and anti-inflammatory properties, which may also contribute to its ability to alleviate anxiety. While more research is needed to confirm these effects, licorice root remains a popular treatment for anxiety in traditional Chinese medicine.

Licorice root is typically consumed as a tea, but it can also be taken in capsule form or added to food. It can be even more effective when combined with other herbs, such as chamomile or lavender. If you are interested in exploring licorice root as a treatment for anxiety, speak to a qualified TCM practitioner to see if it is right for you.

While the fast-paced, constantly hustling society we live in today can be exhilarating, it also takes a toll on our emotional well-being. When our minds are overstimulated with stressors and demands, it can lead to anxiety. However, these natural remedies that have been used for centuries in Traditional Chinese Medicine can help ease anxiety symptoms. If you have anxiety or know someone who does, consider trying some herbal remedies to help ease the symptoms naturally.

Chapter 9

Remedies for Illness

This chapter lists several traditional remedy recipes to cure different illnesses. You'll find user-friendly instructions for preparing teas and other simple concoctions, soups, and restorative meals commonly used in Chinese Herbal Medicine. Before each recipe is a brief explanation for each condition to help you decide for which cases the remedy should be applied.

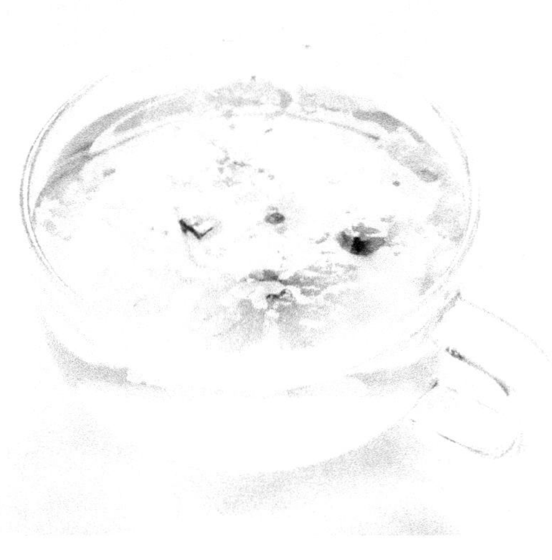

Aloe Vera and Lime Quencher for Stomach Viruses

Stomach viruses are fairly common during summer and typically come with a wide range of symptoms. These include nausea, vomiting, diarrhea, constipation, stomach pain, and fever. Stomach viruses can be caused by several pathogens, which disrupt your gut microbiome and hinder digestion and absorption of food. You need a natural remedy that kills the parasites and restores digestion. Aloe vera, commonly known for its benefits for the skin, is often used in Chinese medicine to treat stomach issues. The following recipe mixes aloe vera gel with limes, creating the perfect combination to relieve stomach issues on a hot summer day.

Here is what you will need:

- 6 limes

- 2 tablespoons of sugar

- 3 ¾ cups of water

- 2 tablespoons of fresh aloe vera gel

- 8 ice cubes, crushed into small pieces

- Lime slices to garnish (optional)

Instructions:

1. Cube the aloe vera gel into tiny pieces and cut the limes in half.

2. Dissolve the sugar in a few tablespoons of water. You can put it in the microwave for a few seconds to speed up this process.

3. Squeeze the juice from the limes, add it to the remaining water and stir the mixture.

4. Prepare the crushed ice in a cup.

5. Pour the sugar water into the lime water, and add the aloe vera gel.

6. Mix everything until well combined, and pour the finished mixture onto the crushed ice.

7. Garnish with lime slices and drink it as soon as possible.

Basil and Garlic Stir Fry for Cold and Flu

Cold and flu are commonly occurring conditions that cause several symptoms of different degrees. These typically affect the respiratory tracts, including cough, stuffed or runny nose, and difficulty breathing. Other symptoms include chills, fever, nausea, loss of appetite, fatigue, and more. Cold and flu are typically caused by viral infections and appear seasonally. According to traditional Chinese medicine practitioners, the best way to treat these illnesses is by drinking plenty of warm liquids, keeping the person warm, and boosting the immune system. However, they also claim that certain herbs and plants in meals can help speed up recovery. This recipe includes basil and garlic - two plants with analgesic, anti-inflammatory, and antioxidant properties.

Here is what you will need:

- 1 pound of shrimp

- 2 tablespoons of vegetable oil

- ⅔ oz of sweet basil, fresh

- 1 teaspoon of black pepper

- 4 garlic cloves

- 1 teaspoon of sugar

- ½ cup of water + 2 additional tablespoons

- 1 tablespoon of cornstarch

Instructions:

1. Prepare the shrimp by shelling, washing, and draining them.

2. Crush the garlic cloves and cut the basil leaves from their stem.

3. Fry the garlic on medium heat for about 2 minutes or until it becomes golden brown.

4. In the meantime, mix the cornstarch with 2 tablespoons of water.

5. Turn the heat to high, add in the shrimp, and continue frying until the shrimp become pink.

6. Add the water, black pepper, basil, and sugar, and cook while stirring for 1 minute.

7. Thicken the shrimp sauce with the cornstarch mixture.

8. Serve with rice or any light dish.

Chive Wine for Small Internal Injuries

Internal injuries, even if they are small and non-life threatening, can be painful. They can also lead to decreased mobility and blood flow, fatigue, feeling cold, and other chronic illnesses. To ensure they heal as fast as possible and won't leave permanent scars, you need a remedy with anti-inflammatory properties, like the one described in the recipe below. This chive wine will also warm you, boosting your circulation and speeding up your recovery.

Here is what you will need:

- 2 ounces of Chinese chives, fresh

- 10 fluid ounces of red wine

Instructions:

1. Bring the red wine to a boil.

2. Cut the chives into tiny pieces and add them to the simmering wine.

3. Let the wine cook with the chives for 5-10 minutes. The longer you leave it, the stronger the infusion.

4. Remove from the stove and let it cool to a temperature comfortable for drinking.

5. Consume while still warm.

Angelica Wine for Poor Blood Circulation

While poor blood circulation is more of a symptom than an actual illness, it can lead to several other symptoms and health issues. It's often caused by poor Qi flow through the body, which is problematic for healthy people and pregnant women. Chinese Angelica is an herb recommended for treating circulatory issues in pregnancy, post-pregnancy, and during menstruation due to its natural health benefits and little-to-no side effects. Besides improving circulation (of blood and Qi), it also helps prevent bleeding and removes blood stagnation.

Here is what you will need:

- 3 ½ ounces of Chinese Angelica

- 2 cups of cognac

Instructions:

1. If the Angelica isn't already sliced, slice it thinly, wash and drain.

2. Pat the slices with the paper towel and wait for a few seconds until they become dry to the touch.

3. Transfer the Angelica slices into a glass container.

4. Pour the cognac over the Angelica slices and leave the mixture steeping in a dark, cool place.

5. Ensure the slices are completely immersed. If not, pour a little more cognac on top of them. It will help prevent mold from developing on top of the slices.

6. Your drink will be ready for consumption after 6 weeks. Consume it whenever you feel it necessary to improve your circulation.

Cardamom and Ginger Tea for Spleen Infection

Spleen infection is a serious condition leading to symptoms like sluggish digestion, diarrhea, vomiting, abdominal pain, fever, and chills. It can also affect the blood and the immune system, as the spleen serves as a reserve tank for blood and lymphocytes crucial for a healthy immune response. Various pathogens can cause spleen infections, but they can be treated with herbs with strong anti-inflammatory properties. Ginger and cardamom are known for their ability to alleviate symptoms of spleen infection.

Here is what you will need:

- 3 ¾ cups of water

- 2 ½ ounces of sugar

- 1 tablespoon of shredded ginger

- 8 pods of green cardamom

- 1 tablespoon of Chinese tea leaves

- 1 ounce of sweet basil

Instructions:

1. Pour the water into a pot, and add the cardamom, sugar, and ginger.

2. Bring to a boil and let it simmer for 10-15 minutes on medium heat. The longer it cooks, the stronger its effect.

3. While the mixture cooks, remove the basil leaves from the fibrous stem and discard the latter.

4. Add the basil leaves to the simmering mixture and cook for 3 more minutes.

5. Remove from the heat, add the tea leaves, and stir to combine.

6. Let the tea steep for 15 minutes, and strain the mixture through a fine sieve or cheesecloth.

7. Transfer the tea to a warm teapot, and drink while still warm.

Pork and Chicken Soup with Buddha's Fruit for Bronchitis

Bronchitis refers to the inflammation of the bronchi, the crucial parts of the lower respiratory tract. The bronchi actively participate in the oxygen-carbon dioxide exchange in the lungs during respiration, and inflammation can lead to breathing difficulties, cough, phlegm, and other symptoms. Bronchitis is typically caused by pathogens invading the lower respiratory tract but can originate from allergies affecting these organs. Bronchitis can lead to asthma and other chronic and acute conditions. A warm, nourishing soup with Buddha's fruit can help alleviate the symptoms and speed up recovery.

Here is what you will need:

- 2 pounds of lean chicken meat

- 1 ounce of pork

- 6 cups of water

- 1 Buddha's fruit

- 1 tablespoon of Chinese wolfberries

- 1 teaspoon of ground black pepper

- 2 teaspoons of salt

- 1 teaspoon of cinnamon

- 1 teaspoon of turmeric

Instructions:

1. Break up the Buddha's fruit, wash, and drain it from the water.

2. Place the chicken, pork, wolfberries, Buddha's fruit, salt, pepper, cinnamon, and turmeric into a pot and cover with water.

3. Bring to a boil, lower the heat, and let it simmer for an hour.

4. Remove the soup from the heat, strain it, and drink it while still hot.

Codonopsis and Astragalus Tea for Heart Issues

Heart conditions can be caused by multiple factors, including congenital, lifestyle, and infection. Due to this, they can manifest through a wide range of symptoms. Some include slow circulation, edema, water retention, excessive perspiration, high blood pressure, and the subjective feeling of being hot or cold all the time. Astragalus roots are very effective in relieving these symptoms. This recipe combines the roots with codonopsis, a plant known for its ability to balance Qi. When the two herbs work together, they help revitalize the body and aid the production of red blood cells while reducing the white blood cell count.

Here is what you will need:

- ½ ounces of codonopsis roots
- ½ ounces of astragalus roots
- 3 ¼ cups of water
- 2 ounces of sugar

Instructions:

1. Rinse and drain the roots.

2. Combine the roots with the sugar and water in a pot and place the pot on the stove.

3. Bring it to a boil, reduce the heat to medium, and let it simmer for 30-40 minutes.

4. Remove from the heat, and strain the tea through a sieve or cheesecloth.

5. Serve according to your preferences. For example, add Chinese dates to sweeten it. Avoid adding sugar.

Mixed Apricot Kernels with Gingko Nuts for Rheumatism

Rheumatism refers to several conditions affecting the joints and the connective tissues. They are followed by inflammation, pain, reduced mobility, and other acute and chronic symptoms. Rheumatic conditions can have several origins, but the most common cause is an autoimmune response, where the immune system reacts to its tissue as a foreign body. The immune response leads to the person's cells attacking the otherwise healthy tissue - in this case, the tissue of the joints and everything around it. The key to relieving the symptoms of rheumatic disorders is applying anti-inflammatory agents like apricot kernels. Also known as Chinese almonds, apricot kernels have a sedative effect and protect the joints from injuries during flare-ups, especially when combined with Ginkgo seeds.

Here is what you will need:

- ⅔ ounces of bitter apricot kernels

- ⅔ ounces of sweet apricot kernels

- 2 ounces of white fungus

- 1 ⅓ ounce of ginkgo nuts

- 4 cups of water

- 5 ounces of sugar

Instructions:

1. Cook the Gingko nuts until they become soft, but not so that you can crush them.

2. Cover the white fungus with water and let it soak some of it up.

3. When it looks like it soaked up plenty of water, rinse, drain, and cut the fungus into bite-sized pieces.

4. Rinse and drain the apricot seeds, and set them aside to dry.

5. When they've dried, combine the seeds with the white fungus, the ginkgo nuts, and water in a pot.

6. Bring the mixture to a boil, lower the heat, and let it simmer for 45 minutes.

7. Stir occasionally, and add water if necessary to prevent the ingredient from burning.

8. After 45 minutes, add the sugar and continue cooking for a few minutes until the sugar has dissolved.

9. Remove from the heat and serve as desired. You can consume it strained while it's hot or wait until it cools down.

Artemisia Tea for Hemorrhoids

Hemorrhoids are a common issue for people with a sedentary lifestyle or a circulatory deficiency. Hemorrhoids are varicose veins (dilated veins with reduced elasticity and circulatory function) that develop in the inner or outer wall of the rectum. They can be accompanied by pain, bleeding, bloody stools, and infection of the affected area. They can also make the passing of the stool more difficult, which aggravates the condition. Artemisia tea can help reduce inflammation and other symptoms, including bleeding from hemorrhoids.

Here is what you will need:

- Chinese tea leaves in the desired amount

- ½ teaspoons of dried artemisia leaves for each cup of tea

- Water as needed

Instructions:

1. Grind the artemisia into a fine or coarse powder. Fine powder will take less time to infuse the water.

2. Place the desired amount of Chinese tea leaves into a pot, add ½ teaspoon of artemisia powder per cup, and cover it with water.

3. Bring the water to a boil, reduce the heat, and let it simmer. The fine powder will only take about 5 minutes to cook, while the coarse variant can take up to 15 minutes.

4. The cooking time also depends on how strong you like your tea. The longer it simmers, the more intense flavor you'll get from the Chinese tea leaves.

5. Remove from the heat, strain, and let it cool a little.

6. Drink as soon as it gets to the temperature you're comfortable consuming.

7. For the best effect, drink one cup of this tea three times a day.

Congealed Tea for Ulcers

Ulcers are sores or small wounds on the stomach lining or the duodenum. They can appear due to stress, overindulgence in spicy food, alcohol, carbonated drinks, medication, infections, and many other reasons. Ulcers cause abdominal pains, nausea, and digestion issues. They can lead to bleeding, bloody vomiting, and bloody stools if perforated. To treat ulcers, the stomach needs to be fortified, and the inflammation in the area reduced, which can be achieved with the appropriate direction of Qi with a simple herbal tea. This recipe is for a Chinese chai tea that will help close the ulcers, moisturize the stomach, and harmonize digestion.

Here is what you will need:

- 1 cup of Chai tea leaves

- 1 cup of sugar

- 3 ½ cups of water

Instructions:

1. Place all the ingredients into a pot, and bring the tea to a boil.

2. After it starts to boil the first time, turn off the heat and let it cool for a few minutes.

3. Once the tea is only slightly warm, bring it to a boil again, and let it simmer for 2-4 minutes.

4. Remove from the heat, let it cool, and strain when it has cooled and settled down.

5. Pour the liquid into a clean container, cover it, and set it aside in a cold and dry place.

6. After 6-12 days, the liquid should have the color of old wine, with a net-like congealed surface. The tea is ready to be consumed if this is the case.

7. Leave it for another 2 days if its surface isn't congealed.

8. Heat the tea slightly before consuming it, and take only 1 spoonful at a time.

9. It can be consumed twice daily - once in the morning and once in the evening.

Walnut and Ginseng Tea for Asthma

While it has a similar etymology as bronchitis, asthma often becomes a chronic condition as opposed to bronchitis, which is typically accompanied by acute respiratory symptoms. Patients with bronchial or allergic asthma often develop symptoms like chronic fatigue and dyspnea (the inability to take large enough breaths for sufficient oxygen supply). They also experience the very characteristic wheezing sound, which often occurs after even the smallest physical exertion. This sound is also accompanied by violent cough attacks due to the increased secretion production in the lungs, fainting, and low blood pressure and saturation levels. This walnut and ginseng tea reduces inflammation, supplements the healthy production of lung tissue, and is an excellent liquid source patients need after a flare-up.

Here is what you will need:

- ¾ cup of sugar

- ⅔ cup of walnuts

- ¼ cup of hawthorn fruit

- 1 teaspoon of ginseng

- 5-6 cups of water

Instructions:

1. Soak the walnuts in cold water for half an hour. Drain and rinse them.

2. Place the walnuts into a pot and pour 5 cups water over them. Blend the walnuts and the water into a thick liquid mixture.

3. Break up the hawthorn fruit, add it to a pot and pour a cup of water over it.

4. Bring it to a boil, let it simmer for 20 minutes, then cool it down. Repeat this 2 more times. Add the ginseng before boiling it for the last 20 minutes.

5. Strain the hawthorn liquid, add the sugar, and let it melt on medium heat, stirring occasionally.

6. Continue stirring while you add the thick walnut liquid and bring the combined mixture to a boil again.

7. Remove from the heat and transfer it into a teapot. You should have a little over 4 cups of concentrated liquid.

8. You can take this tea any time after a flare-up.

Orange Seed and Egg Mask for Inflammatory Skin Conditions

Inflammatory skin conditions, accompanied by acne, redness, itchy, swollen, and dry skin, can be caused by multiple reasons. Food allergies, sensitivity to cleaning agents, and perfume commonly used in body washes and detergents can lead to the skin being inflamed. The conditions can be acute and chronic, with recessive periods and acute flare-ups. In both cases, the symptoms can be treated with an anti-inflammatory agent, which can be applied internally and topically. The latter provides immediate relief for the most prevalent symptoms. The following mask is one of the best examples of these remedies.

Here is what you will need:

- ½ ounces of orange seeds

- 1 egg

Instructions:

1. Separate the egg white from the yolk, and set the latter aside.

2. Grind the orange seeds and combine them with the egg white to get a thick paste.

3. Do an allergy test first on a small patch of skin. If you don't have an allergic reaction, apply the mask to the entire affected area.

4. If you have any redness, pain, or increased itchiness, this remedy won't be a suitable remedy for your condition.

5. This batch makes enough remedy for medium-sized areas (like the face and neck). If you need to cover a larger surface, feel free to adjust the proportions to suit your needs.

These are only a few of the plethora of recipes available for illnesses: research your condition and the associated remedies. Consider the availability of herbs, and always consult your practitioner before committing to a remedy. Although the ingredients are natural, they could have minor side effects, especially if taking pharmaceutical medication.

Chapter 10

Remedies for Pain

Pain is your body's way of alerting you when something is wrong and pointing you in the right direction. However, no one enjoys the uncomfortable and unpleasant sensation it causes. It affects a specific part of the body or the entire body.

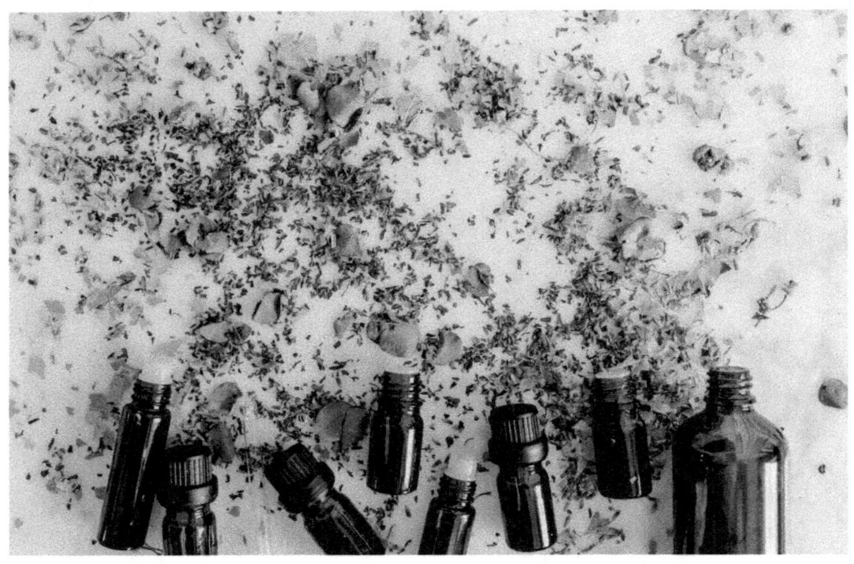

When our nervous system is activated, pain occurs. In other words, we experience pain when our brain interprets the signal sent by nerve fibers. Pain can be sharp, consistent, dull, or short-lived, and it varies depending on its cause or the person's tolerance level.

In many cases, the causes of pain are not implausible. It is caused by a medical condition, injury, or stress from strenuous physical activity. Aside from disorders and chronic illnesses, common causes of pain include headaches, sore throats, muscle cramps, stomach aches, bruises, cuts or burns, and broken bones.

Classification and Causes of Pain

The severity of pain is determined by a person's pain tolerance. Regular headaches become more severe for some people while manageable for others. Although one or more factors cause pain, the various causes have made it easier to classify and treat.

Acute pain is caused by an injury, medical procedure, or illness. It usually occurs suddenly and for short periods, is sharp, and is usually treated in a few days.

A variety of health conditions cause chronic pain, which lasts longer than acute pain and develops over time. They arise from an underlying injury or disease after the initial healing and cause discomfort in the patient. It is also known as functional pain, and because there is no visible injury to the body, it is difficult to identify and restricts daily activities.

Nociceptive pain is caused by bruises, cuts, fractures, or tissue inflammation from osteoporosis or arthritis. While chronic or acute, the main cause is tissue damage, which appears as somatic or visceral pain in the muscles, bones, skin, or internal organs.

Neuropathic pain is caused by nerve damage caused by injury or illness. It could be caused by shingles, cancer, diabetes, or a movement of a spine disc out of place. Neuropathic pain is caused by any activity or injury which puts pressure on the nerve.

Pain is caused by illness, symptoms of illness, chronic diseases, or injury and has crippling effects or changes people's lives. People use medications or therapeutic methods to relieve pain, but in Chinese culture, using herbal medicine or remedies to relieve pain is a common, age-old practice.

Chinese Medicines for Pain Relief

Chinese medicine offers a variety of methods for treating pain, including using herbs and dietary and lifestyle changes. Chinese medicine was popular in earlier eras and is still in demand because nature's gift has been incorporated into the Chinese way of life, diet, and medical practice. It is the cornerstone of their native medical system and is effective for curing a wide range of illnesses.

It treats pain as a reduced or stagnant energy flow, or Qi. The emphasis is on the pain, the area it affects, and how to restore the body to its natural balance because pain depletes the body's energy. Unlike in the Western world, there is no need to administer medications or remedies to alleviate the pain.

The Chinese medicine pharmacopeia, or collection, contains thousands of natural herbs and formulas to restore the body to full functionality. The healing process is centered on how the patient responds to pain relief medications, and the formula is tweaked with each new observation of the patient's progress.

The mediation brings the patient back to normalcy by focusing on the pain or area. The remedy can be in the form of tea, tinctures, oils, or capsules and is carefully prepared with natural healing herbs to improve the health and condition of the person in discomfort.

Chinese medicine relies on natural healing and plant and herb components to help people cope with pain. These herbs and formulas are used singly or synergistically with adequate knowledge of the drug used to comfort and eliminate pain.

Indigenous practices like these might seem complicated or even trivial to the average person, but pain can be overcome by using the natural healing properties of herbs and natural medicine.

The medication is easy to make because it uses herbs grown at home, found in the neighborhood, or purchased at farmers' markets. The herbs are available elsewhere and are not unique to the Chinese. This chapter focuses on traditional pain relievers and the recipes for making them.

Recipes for Remedies That Cure Pain

Chinese herbal painkillers are formulated from various herbs combined for their primary herbal healing properties and synergistic effects or to reduce the side effects of other herbs in the mixture.

How the remedy is given depends on the pain to be relieved, the pain's symptoms, and the person's overall health. It will change over time to accommodate the person's development. The severity of the pain and the amount of herbal treatment the patient can tolerate are additional considerations, but the herb's intended purpose is unaffected.

After cultivating, harvesting, or acquiring the herb from the store, the general practice is to wash and eliminate any dirt or impurity before preparing the herbs into ingestible or applicable forms, and cleaning the herbs aids in achieving a satisfactory level of purity while retaining a high level of potency.

The equipment used in the preparations must be sterilized and cleaned to remove impurities. Most people can't measure how much impurity gets into the mixture when making herbal remedies at home. Still, for the efficacy of the mixture, it's best to follow basic hygiene practices before brewing or preparing an herbal remedy.

Pain in any part of the body is very discomforting, but preparing a pain-reliever mixture gives you a sense of control over your health. Regular painkillers are a quick way to get rid of pain, but with prolonged use, they are rendered useless by natural resistance and could become harmful.

Herbal remedies for pain relief are widely used because they have few or no side effects, are made at home, and have a wide range of curing abilities. Among the most popular herbal remedies for natural pain relief are:

Prunella Vulgaris Tea

Prunella Vulgaris, known as self-heal, is a common herb grown in many parts of the world which has been and continues to be used as a medicinal plant. It is closely related to the mint flower; it grows as a slender purple flower and has a slightly bitter but subtle minty flavor.

Since cooking herbs is similar to preparing a soup, most Chinese remedies come in the form of tea. Prunella Vulgaris tea helps to maintain the body's balance, and, as its name implies, it helps to deal with the pain associated with headaches, wounds, and sore throats.

Dried herbs are harvested or purchased from a local Chinese shop to make a potent Prunella Vulgaris tea. The leaves are thoroughly washed, preferably multiple times, to remove impurities. Modifications or sweeteners are used to adjust the taste to your liking. The taste is recommended to be kept mild, but sweeteners like sweetened winter melon, carrots, sugars, or Chrysanthemum are used to sweeten the taste.

Below are steps to follow in preparing Prunella:

1. Place water in a clean pot and pour in the prunella.

2. Wash, peel, and cut your carrots into sizeable chunks before tossing them into the pot.

3. Allow the mixture to boil and simmer for 30 minutes on a low heat

4. Add your sweetened Winter melon or sweetener of your choice (optional) and boil for 30 minutes.

5. Remove from the heat.

6. Using a strainer, strain your tea into a jug or warm teapot.

7. Serve hot or allow to cool and drink as a cold beverage.

When brewed for longer, the herbs have more time to release their flavors into the liquid, which may account for a later sweetness or bitterness in the beverage. Depending on the intensity of the pain and how frequently it occurs, the tea is consumed daily or less frequently.

Ginseng Tea

Ginseng tea comes to mind first when discussing traditional Chinese medicine for pain relief. Ginseng root is well-known for its use in traditional Chinese medicine and its energy-healing properties. It is used to boost energy and health, in addition to relieving pain, stress, and inflammation. Its health benefits trail has a plethora of applications.

Although available in raw and powdered forms, when brewing ginseng tea, it is strongly advised to use the root or root powder obtained from a reputable ginseng farm rather than ginseng supplements, which might contain pesticides or pose a contamination risk.

To make ginseng tea from ginseng roots, here are steps to take:

1. Clean dried ginseng roots to remove impurities.

2. Pour a cup of water into a pot or kettle and allow to boil. Allowing the water to reach maximum boiling point is required to facilitate the extraction of the compounds (ginsenosides) responsible for ginseng's healing power.

3. Add a variable amount of ginseng roots measuring about 4-5 grams into the water and allow to steep for 15 minutes.

4. Using tongs or a strainer, remove the roots from the tea and leave them to dry on a towel. The root can be reused depending on the duration of the steep and the root size.

5. Add honey to sweeten the taste (optional).

Some of the steps previously mentioned are used to make ginseng tea from ginseng powder.

1. Use ginseng powder or grind the roots to a powder

2. Pour heated water into a cup.

3. Add one teaspoon or a teabag of powdered ginseng root. In most cases, ginseng powder is sold in tea bags.

4. Leave to steep for 3 to 5 minutes, and add honey to taste.

Ginseng is also available in pill form, but it is easier for the body to absorb when consumed as a tea. After drying, the roots are ground into a fine powder and sealed in capsules to make capsules or solid pills. Whether as tea or pills, ginseng is a highly functional herb that helps with pain relief.

Turmeric

Many people only know turmeric as a spice and are unaware of its anti-inflammatory properties. Turmeric is a popular natural treatment for arthritis, inflammation, and joint pain.

Turmeric is a spice, meaning it is used in different ways, such as tea, paste, milk, and food flavoring. One of its constituents (curcumin) is responsible for its pain-relieving properties. The goal of using turmeric alone or combined with other anti-inflammatory spices is to obtain pain-relieving properties.

Turmeric tea is a simple way to consume it. Follow the steps below to make turmeric tea.

1. Measure one teaspoon of turmeric and add four cups of water. (The turmeric can be ground, dried, grated, or powdered, they are all very efficient).

2. Allow to boil for about 10 minutes.

3. Strain the tea and add sweetener to taste.

4. Remove any grains or flakes before drinking.

One of the many ways to consume turmeric is tea. Turmeric is mixed into food or milk, or you can add it to the milk of your choice using the golden milk recipe as a guide. In this liquid milk-based recipe, a teaspoon of turmeric is added to a cup of milk.

You achieve a golden, creamy appearance by adding turmeric to your dairy or dairy-free milk. Black pepper is added to the milk to boost the turmeric effects and hasten its absorption by the body. You can drink the golden milk straight up or use it as a soup and dressing base.

You can incorporate golden milk into your diet by mixing it into your coffee or pouring it over your oatmeal for breakfast. Turmeric is combined with other anti-inflammatory fruits like ginger, berries, banana, and cinnamon to create a delicious anti-inflammatory drink.

Turmeric is used to season foods like chicken or as a dressing for salads and other dishes. It is combined with ginger and carrot to make soup or sprinkled on eggs.

Turmeric is also made into a paste and stored for later use in milk, smoothies, or for preparing cherries. Turmeric paste is a melted blend of spices, black pepper, turmeric powder, and oil:

- A cup of water

- A quarter cup of coconut oil

- One teaspoon of black pepper and freshly grated ginger

- One tablespoon of ground cinnamon

- Half a cup of ground turmeric

Method:
Before adding the oil, add all the powdered ingredients.

Allow to melt after properly mixing with heat until there are no lumps.

Transfer to a jar and store in the refrigerator for later use.

Turmeric is an effective pain reliever, and as a spice, there are numerous ways to incorporate it into our diet and prepare it for consumption. Whatever method you use to prepare it, its pain-relieving properties will be absorbed by your body.

Cinnamon

Despite being a flavoring agent, cinnamon is a natural pain reliever. It's an excellent medicine for arthritic pain. Medically prescribed painkillers help reduce arthritic pain, but cinnamon provides a natural, side-effect-free alternative.

Its active compound, cinnamaldehyde, acts as an anti-inflammatory agent, reducing joint pain and preventing tissue damage, which is a source of pain.

Cinnamon is purchased in its raw form or powder form at the market. It is broken into small pieces and added to soups and other dishes. It is a flavoring in rice dishes, yogurts, curries, and salads.

Follow these steps to prepare your Cinnamon Tea Recipe:

1. Bring water to a boil and pour it into a cup.

2. Add a teaspoon of cinnamon powder and one tablespoon of honey to the cup of hot water.

3. After allowing it to stand for a while, strain the mixture. It is ready to be consumed in the mornings and nights.

Another effective remedy for joint pain is taking a tablespoon of honey and half a teaspoon of cinnamon powder before breakfast. Cinnamon is an effective pain reliever but should not be used carelessly. Take it with caution because too much could cause a migraine.

Myrrh and Frankincense Salve

Myrrh and frankincense are very exotic resins highly valued in many cultures and have a strong aroma. They are difficult to obtain and even more difficult to grind to a powder as they are sold in large chunks.

They are useful for making skin salves and herbal tinctures to treat skin infections and inflammations because of their anti-inflammatory and analgesic properties.

Before making a skin salve with frankincense, myrrh, goldenseal, and cayenne pepper to treat inflammations, prepare an infused oil as a base.

For a sufficient amount of frankincense and myrrh-infused oil, you need half a cup of myrrh and frankincense resins, two tablespoons of cayenne pepper, a quarter cup of goldenseal root, and a few cups of coconut or olive oil. Follow the steps below:

1. Combine powdered frankincense, cayenne pepper, myrrh, and goldenseal root in a mason jar.

2. Fill the jar with oil.

3. Stir the herbs in the jar and add more oil until the herbs are fully submerged in oil.

4. Place the Mason jar in a slow cooker, fill it with warm water until halfway up the jar and place it on low heat.

5. Heat the jar until the oil turns orange. Shake slightly during heating to distribute the herbs in the oil.

6. Before straining, allow the herbs to settle in the oil.

7. Keep the oil after straining it into a clean container for further processing into a skin lotion or salve.

For the preparation of the salve: 4 tablespoons of the already infused oil, one tablespoon of beeswax and shea butter, frankincense, or lavender essential oil (optional). Follow this direction:

1. Using a glass measuring cup and a pan, create a double boiler.

2. Add beeswax, already prepared myrrh and frankincense infused oil, and shea butter into the cup.

3. Turn the double boiler on low heat and simmer the mixture over water until the shea butter and beeswax are melted.

4. Remove the measuring cup and pan from the heat and add the essential oil to the mixture. (Although adding the essential oil into the mixture increases its soothing effects, the salve is still functional without its addition.)

5. Stir the salve with a thin spatula and allow it to cool a little.

6. Pour into tins and seal once the salve is completely cool.

The salve is used to treat skin infections and reduce pain from swelling.

Corydalis

Corydalis is an essential plant in traditional Chinese medicine for relieving pain caused by nerve damage and osteoarthritis. It is widely used by herbalists to treat pain, and because it appears to have no side effects, some consider it the most effective pain reliever after opium.

It has traditionally been used to treat stomach pain, nerve damage, menstrual cramps, and traumatic injuries. Its most concentrated chemical components have a relaxing and relieving effect on the brain.

Corydalis roots are preserved after harvesting for medicinal purposes like tinctures, powders, or teas. To make tea: boil 10g corydalis roots and 3g cinnamon in two cups of water for up to 7 minutes. 5-10g of corydalis powder is dissolved in water and taken twice daily.

To make a corydalis tincture, follow the guide below:

1. Wash and clear the roots of any impurity.

2. Cut and place the root in an airtight jar filled with 20% alcohol and allow it to steep for six or more weeks.

3. Strain to remove the plant parts and package for future use.

For intake, it is advised to add six to twelve drops in water, juice, or beneath the tongue three times a day.

Pain is a very frustrating and incapacitating sensation. It is extremely unpleasant and results from several causes, including injury, illness, or medical procedures. Although regular pain relievers are effective, their cumulative side effects have made the natural alternative of herbal remedy more appropriate.

Traditional Chinese medicine has been used for centuries to treat minor ailments and pain. Instead of a quick fix, natural remedies focus on restoring the body's natural balance and eliminating pain.

A handful of local herbs are brewed, ground, or cooked to create medications for pain relief. Herbs are grown, purchased, and processed using simple recipes. Although side effects are uncommon, taking the potions in moderation is strongly advised, and practicing basic hygiene aids in the reduction of impurities and the preparation of potent medication.

Conclusion

The greatest thing about Chinese Herbal Medicine is that you can put together remedies and techniques tailored to your unique needs. We all have different energies, and bodies are not all made up of the same proportions nor respond to the same things. This is essentially why generic drugs cannot suit everyone and often trigger various side effects.

If you know how to safely create and use herbal formulas, you won't need to worry about experiencing any side effects. All formulas in traditional Chinese medicine incorporate supporting herbs to alleviate possible side effects.

This holistic healing medical system treats the client and not their symptoms. It identifies and targets the root cause of the illness, ensuring long-term wellness and preventing it from returning. Moreover, TCM improves the overall quality of life by improving digestion, treating skin conditions, promoting healthier sleep patterns, and uplifting the patient's mood. You will not experience any more suffering in these areas due to the benefits of this healing system; it is a preventative and boosting method.

Today's fast-paced world leaves everyone feeling on edge. Even the smallest inconveniences can send us into "fight-or-flight" mode, which hinders our mental, physical, and emotional health. TCM helps manage stress more effectively and sends it from a sympathetic nervous state to a parasympathetic healing state.

Now that you have read this book, you know everything about Chinese Herbal Medicine. You've encountered numerous advanced methods and remedies to help treat various ailments and health conditions. However, you shouldn't replace conventional treatment with traditional Chinese medicine, especially if you have serious health problems. Using it as a complementary therapy can help alleviate your symptoms and accelerate healing. You must consult your doctor before using any techniques mentioned in this book, particularly herbology. You don't want your consumed compounds to undermine or react negatively with your prescribed medications.

Upon reading this book, you learned about the history, concepts, and philosophy behind traditional Chinese medicine and gained insight into its different branches. You should be able to tell the difference between Western diagnosis and treatments and TCM diagnosis methods and healing techniques. You've also learned about the main herbs used in Chinese medicine, what and how they're used, their benefits, and what they can help cure.

You must be confident in your abilities before conducting cupping, moxibustion, and herbology techniques. We recommend that you seek the guidance of an experienced practitioner before using these methods on your own. You need to ensure you can safely and effectively conduct these methods. Otherwise, you might not yield the desired results and risk harming yourself or others.

Traditional Chinese medicine has been around for so long, but we have been sucked into modern pharmaceutical concepts. It's time to go back to our roots and traditional medicine. It's time to heal the cause, not the symptoms, leading to a healthier lifestyle and longevity. Reading this book was your first step into a world of natural medicine and remedies and an exciting journey of discovery.

References

Benefits of TCM. (n.d.). Redmint.
https://www.redmint.com/pages/benefits-of-tcm

Chinese medicine. (2019, December 2). Hopkinsmedicine.org.
https://www.hopkinsmedicine.org/health/wellness-and-prevention/chinese-medicine

Chuanxin Wang-OM Clinical / Faculty Supervisor. (n.d.). The Five Vital Substances in Traditional Chinese Medicine (TCM). Amcollege.edu. https://www.amcollege.edu/blog/five-vital-substances-in-tcm

The eight extraordinary meridians: Our genetic imprinting. (2005, December 1). Acupuncturetoday.com.
https://www.acupuncturetoday.com/mpacms/at/article.php?id=30252

The vital substances. (n.d.). Taking Charge of Your Health & Wellbeing. https://www.takingcharge.csh.umn.edu/explore-healing-practices/what-traditional-chinese-medicine/what-qi-and-other-concepts/-vital-substa

Acupuncture & Massage College. (n.d.). Traditional Chinese medicine and lifestyle recommendations. Amcollege.edu. https://www.amcollege.edu/blog/traditional-chinese-medicine-and-lifestyle-recommendations

Batavia, M. (2006). Qigong. In Contraindications in Physical Rehabilitation (pp. 778–782). Elsevier.

Carina. (2008, September 24). TCM Five Element Theory or Wu Xing - Carahealth. Carahealth.com; Carahealth. https://www.carahealth.com/health-articles/traditional-chinese-medicine/five-element-theory-wu-xing

Chinese medicine. (2019, December 2). Hopkinsmedicine.org. https://www.hopkinsmedicine.org/health/wellness-and-prevention/chinese-medicine

Chuanxin Wang-OM Clinical / Faculty Supervisor. (n.d.). Yin-yang in Traditional Chinese Medicine. Amcollege.edu. https://www.amcollege.edu/blog/yin-and-yang-in-traditional-chinese-medicine

Classics of traditional Chinese medicine: Yin and yang. (2001). https://www.nlm.nih.gov/exhibition/chinesemedicine/yin_yang.html

Clayton, V. (2022, July 20). Acupuncture vs. Acupressure: What's the difference? Forbes. https://www.forbes.com/health/body/acupuncture-vs-acupressure/

Deutsche Welle. (2015, August 24). Healthy eating in traditional Chinese medicine. Deutsche Welle. https://www.dw.com/en/healthy-eating-in-traditional-chinese-medicine/a-18619239

Freed, J. (2020, October 23). What is Chinese medicine? American
College of Traditional Chinese Medicine.
https://www.actcm.edu/chinese-medicine

Frost, J. (2018, August 11). The five branches of Traditional
Chinese Medicine. Jenny Dull-Frost.
https://branchesofwellnessacupuncture.com/five-branches-
traditional-chinese-medicine/

Li, M. (2017, October 13). Diet according to Traditional Chinese
Medicine. Royal Treatment Therapeutics.
https://www.royaltreatmenttherapeutics.com/acupuncture/di
et-tcm/

Lifestyle & dietary advice in Chinese Medicine - Geelong Chinese
Medicine Clinic. (n.d.). Com.au.
https://www.geelongchinesemedicine.com.au/services/life-
style-assessment-exercise-advice

The Editors of Encyclopedia Britannica. (2018). Huangdi. In
Encyclopedia Britannica.

The Yellow Emperor - xuanyuan Huangdi - real or myth? - Shen
Yun performing arts. (2016, November 18).
Shenyunperformingarts.org; Shen Yun Performing Arts.
https://www.shenyunperformingarts.org/explore/view/articl
e/e/oRipXNl71aY/yellow-emperor-xuanyuan-huangdi-
chinese-legends

Traditional Chinese Medicine - A brief history. (n.d.).
Villageremedies.com.
https://www.villageremedies.com/blog-articles/traditional-
chinese-medicine-a-brief-history

What is Qi? (and other concepts). (n.d.). Taking Charge of Your
Health & Wellbeing.
https://www.takingcharge.csh.umn.edu/explore-healing-
practices/traditional-chinese-medicine/what-qi-and-other-
concepts

What is Traditional Chinese Medicine? (n.d.). WebMD
https://www.webmd.com/balance/guide/what-is-traditional-
chinese-medicine

Acupuncture, C., & Herbal Clinic. (n.d.). Differences between
TCM and western medicine. China-acupuncture.net.
http://www.china-acupuncture.net/compare.html

Zhang, Q., Zhou, J., & Zhang, B. (2021). Computational
Traditional Chinese Medicine diagnosis: A literature survey.
Computers in Biology and Medicine, 133(104358), 104358.
https://doi.org/10.1016/j.compbiomed.2021.104358

DISHARMONY REVEALED – A CONTEXT FOR HEALING –
The New Chinese Medicine Handbook: An Innovative
Guide to Integrating Eastern Wisdom with Western Practice
for Modern Healing. (n.d.). Doctorlib.Info.
https://doctorlib.info/medical/new-chinese-medicine-
handbook/4.html

Ping Ming Health. (2012, May 27). Chinese medicine diagnosis
(part II): Listening & smelling. Ping Ming Health.
https://www.pingminghealth.com/article/2000/chinese-
medicine-diagnosis-part-ii-listening-smelling/

Acupuncture, & Massage College. (n.d.). What is Qi? Definition of
    Qi in Traditional Chinese Medicine. Amcollege.edu.
    https://www.amcollege.edu/blog/qi-in-traditional-chinese-
    medicine

Chi – what is it? (2018, September 27). Acupuncture That Works.
    https://www.acupuncturethatworks.co.uk/chi-what-is-it/

Chinese medicine. (2019, December 2). Hopkinsmedicine.org.
    https://www.hopkinsmedicine.org/health/wellness-and-
    prevention/chinese-medicine

Chuanxin Wang-OM Clinical / Faculty Supervisor. (n.d.). Yin-yang
    in Traditional Chinese Medicine. Amcollege.edu.
    https://www.amcollege.edu/blog/yin-and-yang-in-
    traditional-chinese-medicine

The meridians —. (n.d.). Rising Moon Tai Chi.
    https://www.risingmoontaichi.net/the-meridians

Abdur-Rahim, Y. (2018, October 1). Facial cupping: How it works,
    benefits, side effects, and more. Healthline.
    https://www.healthline.com/health/facial-cupping

Clark, N. (2016, August 24). Gua Sha vs. Cupping – Which one is
    better? Sidekick Blog | Unlocking Movement; Sidekick
    Blog. https://blog.sidekicktool.com/gua-sha-vs-cupping-
    which-one-is-better/

Different types of gua Sha tools you should know about. (2021,
    May 18). Supergreat.com.
    https://supergreat.com/articles/gua-sha-tools

Hampton Wick Health. (2019, December 7). Tuina, Cupping & Gua Sha - What is it? —. HAMPTON WICK HEALTH. https://www.hamptonwickhealth.com/hwhblog/2019/11/5/tuina-cupping-amp-gua-sha-what-is-it

James, A. (2021). Cupping Therapy: A Complete Guide on the benefits of cupping therapy to heal muscle and body pains, prevent injuries and reduce inflammation. Independently Published.